Dental Benefits and Practice Management

Dental Benefits and Practice Management

A Guide for Successful Practices

EDITED BY

Michael M. Okuji, DDS, MPH, MBA

Dental Director
Delta Dental of Colorado
Denver, Colorado, USA

WILEY Blackwell

This edition first published 2016 © 2016 by John Wiley & Sons, Inc.

Editorial Offices

1606 Golden Aspen Drive, Suites 103 and 104, Ames, Iowa 50010, USA

The Atrium, Southern Gate, Chichester, West Sussex, PO19 8SQ, UK

9600 Garsington Road, Oxford, OX4 2DQ, UK

For details of our global editorial offices, for customer services and for information about how to apply for permission to reuse the copyright material in this book please see our website at www.wiley.com/wiley-blackwell.

Authorization to photocopy items for internal or personal use, or the internal or personal use of specific clients, is granted by Blackwell Publishing, provided that the base fee is paid directly to the Copyright Clearance Center, 222 Rosewood Drive, Danvers, MA 01923. For those organizations that have been granted a photocopy license by CCC, a separate system of payments has been arranged. The fee codes for users of the Transactional Reporting Service are ISBN-13: 978-1-1189-8034-7/2016.

Library of Congress Cataloging-in-Publication Data

Dental Benefits and Practice Management : A Guide for Successful Practices / [edited by] Michael M. Okuji.
    p. ; cm.
  Includes bibliographical references and index.
  ISBN 978-1-118-98034-7 (pbk.)
I. Okuji, Michael M., editor.
[DNLM: 1. Insurance, Dental–United States.   2. Insurance Benefits–United States.
3. Practice Management, Dental–United States. W 260 AA1]
  HG9391.5.U6
  368.38′2300973–dc23
                       2015036762

A catalogue record for this book is available from the British Library.

Wiley also publishes its books in a variety of electronic formats. Some content that appears in print may not be available in electronic books.

Cover image: Jumpeestudio/457707001/Getty Images

Set in 9/12pt Meridien by SPi Global, Pondicherry, India
Printed and bound in Malaysia by Vivar Printing Sdn Bhd

1   2016

About the author

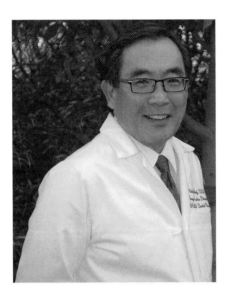

Michael M. Okuji is the Dental Director at Delta Dental of Colorado. He maintained a private practice in San Francisco, California, and was a Group Practice Director at the University of California, Los Angeles. He is the editor and cowriter of the book *Dental Practice: Get in the Game* (2010) and the cowriter of the 12-part web course "Practice Administration" for the NYU Lutheran Dental Medicine.

Contents

List of contributors

Matthew Cassady, JD
Compliance Director, Delta Dental of Colorado, Denver, USA

Gary Herman, DDS, FACD
Supervising Group Practice Director, School of Dentistry, University of California,
Los Angeles, USA

Dennis Lewis, DDS
President and CEO, Dental Aid, Inc., Louisville Colorado, USA

David Okuji, DDS, MBA, MS
Associate Director, Pediatric Dentistry, NYU Lutheran Dental Medicine, Brooklyn, USA

Preface

This book is written at a time when the world of dental practice is under stress. The high cost to deliver dental care under fee ceilings with new entrants in the delivery system rends the very fabric of the solo private practice that dentists cherish. Dentists struggle to maintain this dental care delivery system that served them well against external economic and social pressure. The economic stress comes from the rising cost to run the mom-and-pop dental store, embarrassingly high student debt, and capped reimbursement rates. The social pressure arises from the large number of consumers with no dental benefits, federal dental benefits, and private dental benefits that cannot access affordable dental care and the lack of a transparent and accountable health processes with outcome metrics. The story of stress from an external force is similar to the US automotive industry in the 1960s when Detroit was convinced that American cars were the best in the world and that Americans treasured these tail-finned wonders so much that they would never abandon their American beauties for small, plain, and inexpensive cars manufactured outside of Detroit. After much loss, anguish, and bailouts, Detroit changed in order to survive, and so must dentistry change to remain relevant.

The book is divided into three main sections: (1) the history of dental insurance; (2) dental claim system; and (3) competitive strategies. The first section is the history of dental benefits and how we got to today's dental benefit system. The section points out that while every living practicing dentist has only experienced a reimbursement milieu that is private and employer centered, it has not always been so nor is it how it is fated to be tomorrow. The second section is how to effectively and efficiently work within the dental benefit claim system to become streamlined and patient centered in an ethical and legal manner. The third section seeks solutions to accessible and accountable dental care delivery as it peers into the future of dental benefits and how the different constituents in the system can position themselves for a competitive advantage.

Chapter 1, "Why dental benefits?," is the history of dental benefits, as we know it today, beginning in the mid-20th century as consumers gain prepaid dental care coverage through unions and employers. More consumers begin to access dental care, and the solo practice of private practice dentistry blossomed into full flower. Dentists moved up the financial pecking order from being a Chevrolet to a Mercedes-Benz. In the 21st century, the Patient Protection and Affordable Care Act is the end product of the unsustainable growth of health-care costs that leaves too many without access to basic dental care. During the period of growth of dental care benefits, the cost to receive dental care rises to the point that fewer consumers can afford dental care even when they possess dental benefits.

The stress introduced into the system to the provider, consumer, payer, and government becomes the tipping point for reflection and fundamental change in the system. The question remains as to who will foment change to shape tomorrow's dental care delivery system.

Processing the dental benefit claim and creating the streamlined and patient-centered practice become a critical issue as the principal method for dental care delivery, the solo private practice, comes under increasing stress to cope with the financial and systematic burden placed upon it. It's for relevance and financial survival that the solo private practice embraces the systems presented in Chapter 2, "Dental benefits: Get it done"; Chapter 3, "Dental benefits: Get it right"; Chapter 4, "Patient-centered practice"; and Chapter 5, "Streamlined dental practice."

What is clear is that economic and social change is upon us and the current model of dental practice must change too or dentists become irrelevant to the process. Chapter 6, "Patient Protection and Affordable Care Act," describes the landmark legislation that changes health-care financing and health-care delivery; Chapter 7, "Ethics and ethical behavior," frames the dental profession's challenge to remain grounded and true during change; and Chapter 8, "Stay out of trouble," describes the consequence of making self-centered choices for personal gain.

The solutions proffered in Chapter 9, "Analysis to action," are for both short-term and long-term competitive strategy. Those practitioners with 5 years remaining in a career can incorporate the short-term solutions and thrive. The Thomas Swain model is introduced where a practitioner, 35 years into practice, takes a baby step to be in control of his future. Chapter 9 further speaks to practitioners with a 10-year or more professional practice horizon who are best served to recast their current operating model and begin to think in terms of a networked system. To work in a networked system whose input and output are measured, transparent, and accountable is a formidable hurdle for the dentists who selected the profession in order to own their own independent business and who are trained to do procedures without oversight. But there are solutions for the dentist. Detroit changed itself in a painful transition to a lower-cost, reliable product to regain its competitive edge. And so must dentists reposition themselves to the competitive models.

Dental care delivery and dental care financing had many possible paths to take in the past 60 years. The paths chosen were financially beneficial to the dental profession but left too many people unable to access affordable basic dental care. To cope with the stress of today's dental care delivery system, tomorrow's system will continue to change to address and accommodate the needs of our society as a whole not just the dental profession. The change will accelerate at such a rapid pace that the prudent practitioner needs to assiduously prepare today to remain relevant. To sit on the sideline and wait for the golden age to return is a fool's errand. Today's dental school graduate can never hope to practice in a small, solo, and independent practice as I did in the 1980s.

This book is written as the personal view of each contributor. The book is not a dispassionate historic review but rather a perceived preview of a future state. The content is not presented as new knowledge but rather the distillation of knowledge and observation of the system that forms an opinion. As such, the interpretations and solutions to dental benefit administration, practice management, and dental care delivery are open to alternate interpretation and forecast.

My hope is that the book provokes thoughtful discussion on the role of dentists and dentistry in health care and guides the readers to successfully position themselves to serve as a critical cog in the new health-care system and continue to thrive and prosper. For however much we wish it to be, the path for dentists and dental care delivery does not portend status quo ante.

Acknowledgments

This book could not have been written without the expertise, insight, and gift of time generously given by the contributors to complete this project. Their insight lent the personal nature of the manuscript.

I am forever indebted to two formidable mentors who framed my worldview. Max H. Schoen of the University of California, Los Angeles, introduced me to the quantitative nature of dental care delivery and finance. Clifton O. Dummett of the University of Southern California guided me to look into the human spirit for inspiration in all my endeavors. Both had visions of the potential of health-care delivery to serve the whole community that transcended the parochial status quo ante of their time. They are giants among men and I miss them so.

I also would like to thank Rick Blanchette of Wiley Blackwell for his confidence and patience in the production of this book. He took my concept and gave it wings. My heartfelt appreciation goes to Lilit Mazmanyan who provided invaluable assistance with many details of the manuscript and with her gentle prodding enabled me to complete the project.

PART I
History of Dental Insurance

CHAPTER 1

Why dental benefits?

Michael M. Okuji

Delta Dental of Colorado, Denver, USA

Introduction

This chapter delves into the history of dental benefits and lays the groundwork for the subsequent chapters. The story is one of the social transformations of health care in the USA and the expansion of access to care to wider segments of our society. Prepaid dental benefits available to a worker and their family did not exist, in the way we understand dental benefits, until the last half of the 20th century. From that point in the 1950s to the new millennium, dental benefits broadened in scope and depth as coverage grew to include new eligible members. Dental benefits that became available to a wide swath of consumers profoundly changed the dental profession and dental care delivery.

Dentists enjoy a great deal of professional autonomy and independence in their practice. These features attracted generations of students into the profession and shaped their dental personality to the point the dentistry is rated the number one best job in the USA. From the mid-20th century, the emergence of dental benefits fueled the demand for dental services that fostered dental practice growth and lifted the dentist into the club of well-paid professionals. This is the world into which all dentists who practiced at the turn of the 21st century were born.

But the health-care world continues to evolve into a new order from care delivered by guilds to fraternal group purchases, to industry and union-provided health care, to capitated care, to the emergence of dental benefit companies to the Affordable Care Act. Now, dentists must once again adapt to a profound change in the order of dental care delivery to continue to deliver quality care to a wider segment of the population.

This chapter sets the stage for the coming chapters. Perspective is important to understand that change in the way dental care is delivered and financed has changed over the past 150 years and will continue to change. The status quo isn't destiny.

Dental Benefits and Practice Management: A Guide for Successful Practices, First Edition.
Edited by Michael M. Okuji.
© 2016 John Wiley & Sons, Inc. Published 2016 by John Wiley & Sons, Inc.

The coming of health insurance

We all practice and thrive in a world where dental benefits are a common benefit of employment. We have always practiced where patients we targeted for care had access to dental benefits. While we sometimes struggle with the administrative requirements to bill for our services and chafe at the paper work and the rules of the road, we understand that dental benefit coverage drives patients to our offices. Without dental benefits, many people would not seek dental care on a regular basis and dentists would struggle to fill chairs. For those dentists that started dental practice in the 1960s around new housing developments in the former fruit orchards of the Santa Clara Valley (CA) that became Silicon Valley, the convergence of employer-purchased dental benefits with families moving to new homes proved to be a true golden age to start from scratch a solo private practice and grow a patient base at a lightning-fast pace. So for many dentists, dental benefits proved to be godsend for their practice and their patients.

But dental benefits are a relatively new phenomenon and health insurance didn't always exist. Can you imagine a world where all of your medical, hospital, and prescription bills are paid out of pocket? Can you imagine a world where the middle class pays a large proportion of their income for a medical bill? Can you imagine a world where the working poor are consigned to welfare infirmaries?

The manner in which health care is paid evolved slowly in the USA over the past 150 years. Historically, medical care was available to and paid by principally the upper class with the hospital portion of care taking place in their home. Only the poor went to a hospital. The middle class and the working poor were left to seek episodic care at rates that comprised a significant portion of their income. The very poor sought care at charity infirmaries.

In the 19th century, on the East Coast, fraternal organizations and benevolent societies sprang up among the immigrant tenements to help pay for health care through the voluntary, mutual pooling of money. The fraternal organizations contracted with individual medical providers to deliver care on a prepaid per-capita basis. This medical financing arrangement was more prevalent on the East Coast than out West because of the high density of immigrant populations on the East Coast. Young physicians struggling to establish a private practice contracted on the prepaid basis with these groups for their services but hurriedly left the arrangement as fast as they could once their private practice grew. Organized medicine, in the form of the local medical society, frowned on prepaid contract medical care and ostracized these young and struggling physicians that participated in such arrangements and often refused their membership into the medical society. Out on the West Coast, a large French immigrant community in San Francisco established a French hospital, La Societe Francaise de Bienfaisance Mutuelle, during the gold to aid their French compatriots.

Early in the 20th century, industries like the railroad and mining established health centers for their employees. Industry medical care was limited to work-related injuries to get the workers back to the job. The railroads hired physicians along their rail lines to care for their workers. In the mining industry, unions hired physicians to care for those with injuries from mining accidents. Throughout this period, tension existed among industries, unions, organized medicine, and the government on the proper role of health insurance in the American society and on the people who would control payments to hospitals and physicians. For physicians, it was about the autonomy of the medical profession from any outside influence over who and what controls the cost of care and where it is controlled. For industries, unions, and the government, it was also about the cost of care and gaining access to care for a wider swath of the population.

With the coming of the Depression, workers' wages plummeted or disappeared all together. Hospital and medical visits decreased and physician bills were left unpaid so that families could pay for their food and rent. During the Depression, medical care became recognized as an essential welfare need, and welfare agencies began to pay physicians for their medical services. While the government-sponsored medical relief fund was a benefit to the lower-paid physicians, organized medicine urged all of its members to hold the line against any form of medical insurance. Third-party payment for physician services was seen as the first step toward the socialized medicine and the loss of professional autonomy. The response of organized medicine, in the form of the American Medical Association and its constituent medical societies, to the financial crisis on young physician income, brought on by the Great Depression, was to limit the physician supply (limit medical student spaces in medical school) and increase the price of medical care (through physician autonomy) rather than stimulate the demand for physician services through health insurance. Autonomy and high fees trumped more patient access to medical care.

Since the turn of the 19th century, physician autonomy has been a recurring theme from the medical profession. The issues of the dentist supply (too many), dentist autonomy (organized dentistry over consumers), and the financing and delivery of health care (status quo) are as fresh today as they were 100 years ago. These issues are not a new, unique 21st-century phenomenon, and the response from the dental profession to the financing of and access to health care is the same. The difference that drives change that didn't exist 100 years ago is the Internet with disseminated health information, changing consumer purchasing behavior, and the advent of the Affordable Care Act (Chapter 6).

Private health insurance

In the 1930s, simultaneously, as Franklin Roosevelt's Social Security legislation to support the elderly was born, his national health insurance efforts died. The American Medical Association's campaign to paint national health insurance as socialized medicine was too powerful to overcome. But, following the Second World War, national health insurance was once again resurrected and hotly contested but three times defeated even though President Harry Truman was a strong proponent of a single universal health insurance plan. The thrice-defeated effort to establish a national health insurance program meant that health insurance in America would remain a private enterprise rather than a government program. The question then became, "Who in the private would control health insurance? Would it be a commercial enterprise or the medical profession?" The form of private health insurance would take different changing forms in the next 60 years.

Dental insurance is designed to provide financial assistance for events that are relatively high frequency, low cost, and predictable. Many patients have a general sense of their oral health status that allows them to work with their dentist in regard to the course of their treatment.

In dentistry, there are a high number of alternative treatments and materials from which to choose, each with its own set of cost, benefit, and risk. The essence of solo private practice allows treatment decisions to be developed ad hoc, independent of the peer oversight as would occur in a hospital or physician group practice. Treatment decision is considered the prerogative of the dentist as determined by the rule of what-is-effective-in-my-hands standard of care that can be at odds with the dental professions body of knowledge and evidence-based care.

However, dental treatment can usually be postponed, sometimes for years, and that creates a high potential for adverse selection. Those without coverage may "store up" needed care until they are covered by dental insurance. As a result, a well-designed insurance plan creates incentives for subscribers to remain in the plan for a long time.

Moral hazard

Insurance requires the insurer to assume a financial risk. It derives a gain when it estimates utilization accurately and sustains a loss when it does not estimate utilization accurately. Too much gain and competitors enter the field that drives the price to the consumer down. Too much loss and the company is out of business.

A moral hazard is a lack of incentive to guard against risk knowing that one is protected from its financial consequence by insurance. The presence of insurance, itself, can lead to moral hazard and cause increased loss. Insurance requires that an insured risk and the loss that ensues is unambiguous when it occurs and beyond the control of the insured. Otherwise, the insurer cannot estimate their probable cost of care. Difficulty arises in underwriting dental plans because dental disease is not always a well-defined condition, the course of treatment is not codified, and many of the costs of treatment are within the control of the insured and the provider. So, dental benefit plans, like all insurance, must control for moral hazard.

An insurance company incurs moral hazard when the insured is insulated from financial risk of the care and the provider controls the cost of that care, the case where the provider says you need it, the patient says I want it, and both say someone else should pay for it. Moral hazard is exacerbated when the provider of the care works in isolation away from the scrutiny of other providers and there is no clear, evidence-based solution for a particular diagnosis as in dentistry. Moral hazard exists when treatment selection ambiguity exists and both the insured and the provider are insulated from the consequences of the cost of care.

In group insurance, all subscribers have the opportunity to benefit from pooled community resources and utilization risk. Sometimes, an opportunity appears for an individual to benefit from temporary personal advantage to overuse resources. When an individual continually takes advantage of the common good, the system fails and shuts down. The fix to the problem of moral hazard is to spend resources to identify and control those that take more from the community good. The mechanisms to pay to enforce the rules are like taxes to pay the police and water meters to control water waste. Investing in the public good is good if moral hazard can be controlled. Transparency controls moral hazard.

Moral hazard gives the free rider an increased benefit at the expense of the other members of their risk group. The unrestrained opportunity for a free rider to disregard financial expense increases the cost for the entire risk group and the free rider needs to be restrained in order to keep costs down for the whole group. To do so, private insurance evolved into three types of plan designs defined by the benefit they delivered and the method to control moral hazard. The insurance plan design types are indemnity insurance, benefit service plan, and direct service. Each party benefits from certain elements of a plan design.

Indemnity insurance

Indemnity plan design is fee for service that reimburses the subscriber directly for costs incurred although the bill is not usually paid in full. The subscriber is free to choose any willing provider and the provider is free to charge their patient any fee. Indemnity plan design allows a provider to price discriminate among patients and charge more to some and less to others. The what-the-market-will-bear design allows the provider to apply the wallet x-ray. The patient pays the medical bill when the expense is incurred and then submits a claim that is paid directly to the subscriber.

The indemnity insurance plan design creates the least interaction between the practitioner and the payer. The payer assumes little or no responsibility to their subscriber for the cost or the quality or quantity of care. The insurance plan controls for moral hazard through the application of a deductible amount, cost share, and a benefit maximum that constrains the member's tendency to become a free rider and disregard the financial consequences of their choice.

Dentists prefer that dental insurance be indemnity insurance. Indemnity insurance does not require the dentist enter into any agreement with the insurer. Rather, the indemnity insurer has an agreement with the insured where payments are submitted and reimbursed by and to the insured. The dentist is not held to any specific fee and is free to choose the type, intensity, and frequency of treatment. Dentists collect for their services on a fee-for-service, per-piece basis and are free to price discriminate among patients. This relationship creates the ample opportunity for moral hazard. There are virtually no pure dental indemnity plans in existence today.

Benefit service plan

Benefit plans offer employers a dental product with certain guarantees for their employees. Plan design is fee for service that guarantees payment directly to the provider and sometimes covers the service in full for diagnostic and preventive services. This is where the similarity to dental indemnity insurance ends.

The participating panel of credentialed dentists is the defining element of a benefit plan design. To offer this feature, the benefit plan actively enrolls and credentials dentists into a panel of participating providers. Providers enter into a participating provider agreement with the benefit company that contractually defines their relationship to each other and the provider's obligation to the subscriber.

A benefit plan offers subscribers certain maximum fee guarantees when they seek care from a participating provider. This is a significant feature for the subscriber because the comparative cost of a health-care service, unlike other kinds of consumer services, is opaque to the consumer and the knowledge imbalance in favor of the provider can lead to provider-induced demand. Providers sometimes decry this maximum fee because every patient is reimbursed at same fee level that restricts the provider's ability to use a sliding fee scale among patients. Both indemnity and benefit plans attempt to control overutilization of services (the moral hazard) through a waiting period, deductible, frequency, limitation, and exclusion features of the plan design.

The dental benefit plan can be a risk plan where the benefit company assumes the financial risk for the utilization of services or an administrative service only plan where the employer retains the financial risk for the utilization of services and the benefit company provides the services to administer the plan. In both instances, the benefit plan offers the subscriber access to a panel of participating dentists.

The first dental benefit plans, like the Washington Dental Service, paid for dental services like an indemnity insurer but was actually a dental benefit service plan. It is more accurate to say that a dental benefit plan is more liberal in its fee, policy, and procedure than other benefit plans.

Direct service plan

Direct service plan designs combine both the benefit and the delivery of care. That is, a direct service plan collects prepayment from the payer (employer or individual) and also directly delivers the care through its own panel of dentists. The direct service plan is responsible for the cost, quantity, and quality of the service. Kaiser Permanente is an example of a direct service plan design. Kaiser Permanente arose from the work of Sidney Garfield's industrial programs in construction (Colorado River Aqueduct Project and The Grand Coulee Dam) and shipyards (Kaiser Shipyards). The projects paid Garfield a fixed payment for each worker in return for all medical services. Kaiser Permanente began to accept public enrolment in 1945 with the support of the International Longshoremen's and Warehousemen's Union and the Retail Clerks Union.

One early dental direct service plan was Max Schoen's Harbor Dental Group (Los Angeles County, California) in the 1950s. Like Kaiser Permanente, Schoen's dental group worked with the International Longshoremen's and Warehousemen's Union and the Pacific Maritime Association (ILWU-PMA) and the Retail Clerk's Union. Schoen initially treated the children of union members on a per-member per-month benefit plan. With its focus on prevention, the Harbor Dental Group realized higher utilization of preventive care and lower extraction rate than other dental plan designs as Schoen recounts in his 1969 UCLA doctoral dissertation. However, Schoen's practice model that was fixed fee and closed panel found little support among private practitioners and organized dentistry that favored fee-for-service payment with freedom to choose a dentist. As with similar plan designs in the past, Schoen's model was characterized as socialized health care that challenged the autonomy of dentists and was to be avoided at all costs. A successful direct service plan posed stiff competition to the solo fee-for-service model.

Despite opposition by and ostracism from the dental association, Schoen's Harbor Dental Group continues to thrive to this day and Max went on to an illustrious career in academia and health services research. The principles that Schoen championed 60 years ago are the same principles embedded within the current accountable care organization (ACO) models. ACOs supported by the Affordable Care Act foster a shift to Schoen's direct service plan model that is focused on disease prevention, patient focus, cost-effective care, disease management, and health outcome. The Harbor Dental Group enabled children to access care that improved dental health in a cost-efficient manner 50 years before the Berwick introduced the Triple Aim to health-care reform. It appears that what's old is new again.

Direct reimbursement

In the dental reimbursement market, a direct reimbursement plan is a permutation of an indemnity plan where the subscriber has a set benefit amount available to use for care and the provider decides the quantity and cost of that care. The presence of moral hazard exists for the member and especially for the provider when the entire fee is paid upon the asking with nothing to control the fee or the quantity of services. The direct reimbursement plan design is probably the most expensive plan for the employer, the payer, to maintain.

Health insurance: The Blues

In response to third-party arrangements for hospital payment by commercial private parties, physicians sought to control both the financing and the delivery of medical care.

For over a century, fraternal organizations, mutual benefit societies, industries, unions, and employers developed prepaid programs in order to mitigate the cost of medical care, hospitalization, disability, and death. Immigrant groups formed mutual benefit organizations to insure against loss of wages due to illness and death.

These initial efforts to control health-care costs to a group were local and limited in scope. On a larger scale, industries and unions developed medical service plans to protect their workers against compensable on the job injury. When mutual benefit groups, unions, or companies contracted or directly hired physicians on a capitated basis to deliver medical services to their group, organized medicine vehemently opposed the prepaid arrangement on the grounds that this third-party relationship infringed upon proper medical care. But as these types of pre-payment arrangements continued to grow in number and scope, physicians sought to control the process.

The Blues are two physician-led health service companies with considerable influence on prepaid health care. Blue Cross is the older sibling that provided hospital benefits. The birth of Blue Cross took place in 1929 when Baylor University Hospital provided 1500 schoolteachers prepaid hospital care benefits. Baylor soon offered the same hospital coverage to thousands of other people as the hospital plan expanded to other hospitals in the area and to other states. Group hospitalization payment opened the floodgate to the acceptance of health insurance for medical care. Blue Shield, the physician's shield, provided medical benefits.

Physicians approved of the Baylor hospital plan because during the Depression, the plan paid the hospital bill and left cash for their patients to pay their medical bill. But physicians worried about applying the same principle of hospital insurance to medical services. The thought of third-party payment for medical services, even if it meant more income for young physicians, was anathema to the established physicians. The thought of the third-party payer, even a physician lead payer, was perceived as a threat to physician autonomy and hegemony over medical care.

Never the less, in 1939, a statewide medical benefit plan appeared in California sponsored by the California Medical Association and was called the California Physicians Service, the physician's shield. This medical benefit plan paid its physicians as if it were an indemnity plan with fee for service at the physician's retail fee. Similar medical benefit plans were established in Michigan, New York, and Pennsylvania. Blue Shield (medical service) and its older sibling Blue Cross (hospital service) cooperated to control the hospital and medical benefit market to dampen commercial insurer competition and to keep the commercial insurance companies incursion into health insurance at bay. The two Blues worked in different ways. Blue Cross was more of a prepayment model and offered service benefits. Blue Shield followed an insurance model and allowed physicians to apply a sliding scale to their fees to charge some patients more than others. Today, the Blues continue to provide both hospital and medical benefits.

Federal health benefits

When President Lyndon Johnson signed Medicare into law at the Harry S. Truman Library on July 30, 1965, he told the nation that it had all started with the man from Independence. Truman, Johnson said, had planted the seeds of compassion and duty that led to the enactment of Medicare, a national health insurance for the aged through an expanded Social Security system.

Truman was the first president to publicly endorse a national health insurance program. As a senator, Truman became alarmed at the number of draftees who had failed their induction physicals during the Second World War. For Truman, these rejections meant that the average citizen could not afford to visit a physician to maintain their health. Truman said that is all wrong in his book and tried to fix it so the people in the middle-income bracket can live as long as the very rich and the very poor.

Truman's first proposal in 1945 provided for physician and hospital insurance for working aged workers and their families. A federal health board was to administer the program with the government retaining the right to fix the fees for service, and doctors could choose whether or not to participate. This proposal was defeated after, among many factors, the American Medical Association labeled the president's plan socialized medicine that took advantage of the public's concern over communism in Russia.

Truman was never able to create a national health-care program. He was able to draw attention to the country's health needs, legislated for funds to construct hospitals, expand medical aid to the very poor, and provide for the expansion medical research. In honor of his continued advocacy for national health insurance, Johnson presented Truman and his wife Bess with Medicare cards Number 1 and Number 2 in 1966.

The federal government did become a major health insurer when the Great Society of President Lyndon Johnson established two groundbreaking programs: Medicare for older adults and Medicaid for the poor and disabled. Up to this point in time, the federal government played little role in health-care insurance. The 1965 Medicare legislation established the precedent for government to participate in the health-care financing for its citizens. In 1967, the Early Periodic Screening, Diagnosis, and Treatment (EPSDT) program was established and marked the first mandate for pediatric Medicaid benefits. The purpose of EPSDT was to provide comprehensive and preventive health care for children under 21 years old by eliminating economic barriers to health care. The 1989 Omnibus Budget Reconciliation Act required that dentists rather than physicians perform EPSDT dental screenings with the effect that children were funneled into the dental care system.

Later, in 1997, the State Children's Health Insurance Program (SCHIP) extended coverage to the children of working poor families who did not qualify for Medicaid benefits. When SCHIP expired in 2007, the program was reincarnated as the Children's Health Insurance Program Reauthorization Act (CHIPRA) when President Barack Obama signed it into law in 2009.

CHIPRA underlies many of the precepts of the Patient Protection and Affordable Care Act (ACA) in that it mandates dental benefits for children and adolescents, establishes a new definition of dental care, and addresses the issues of prevention, workforce, quality, reporting, and the dental safety net. The ACA exemplifies a deep commitment of President Obama and his legislative supporters to make health care available to vulnerable populations defined by age, socioeconomic status, or health condition. This commitment is demonstrated by mandated dental care for children, dental education programs for underserved populations, and promotion of new classes of dental care providers to serve those with limited access to dental care.

The Patient Protection and Affordable Care Act, Medicaid, and CHIPRA represent major and lasting efforts of the federal government to influence and extend health-care benefits to the entire population.

Dental benefits

As late as 1960, the percentage of personal dental care expenditures in the USA covered by health insurance or some form of third-party payment was so small as to be reported as zero. Families accessed dental care as needed. During this period, full dentures were common even among the middle class and dentists were adept at fabricating removable appliances to replace extracted teeth. The loss of adult teeth at an early age was accepted as the natural progression of age. During this period, dentist income was modest, more Buick than Cadillac.

However, a profound change in dental care utilization was on the horizon. On the West Coast, a major stimulant to dental benefits occurred in 1954 when the ILWU-PMA established a children's dental program. Two group practices contracted with the ILWU-PMA to provide dental services on a capitated basis in port cities of San Francisco and Los Angeles. After the successful introduction of the ILWU-PMA pilot program, there was a steady growth of third-party payment plans. Throughout the 1960s, access to dental insurance offered families a new employment benefit that increased the number of members who sought dental care. A dental benefit is nonwage compensation for the employee and a tax deduction for the employer. With the growth of dental benefit membership and the increased ability to access dental care, dentist's financial stature grew beyond that of their predecessors as liberal dental benefits drove families to seek dental care and dentist incomes grew year upon year. This firmly boosted the dentist into the upper middle class to where Mercedes-Benz is now organized dentistry's endorsed automobile.

The function, design, and implementation of dental care benefits continue to evolve as dentists, dental organizations, government payers, commercial insurers and the public struggle to balance the cost, quality, access, and equity of health care across a wide and deep spectrum of need.

Dental service company

In the 1950s, to thwart commercial insurance incursion into dental benefits, the state dental associations in Washington, Oregon, and California established dental service corporations like the physician-sponsored health benefit companies, the Blues. The new dental service corporations in these three states provided dental care benefits to the ILWU-PMA pilot program with a design of open panels and fee-for-service reimbursement. Dentists sensed the opportunity to gain access to a new patient base, be paid fee for service at their retail fee, control the dental benefit market, and keep commercial dental plans at bay. With agreement from the Washington State Dental Association, the Washington State Dental Service Corporation (WSDSC) was created in 1954. In the ensuing 20 years, WSDSC pioneered the dental benefit industry and subsequently broadened and grew the dental benefit industry segment into emergency coverage for children, adult dental coverage, and added dental benefit contracts with the Boeing Company and the Washington Education Association. The Federal Trade Commission soon had concern over dentists controlling both the benefit payment and delivery of care to the detriment of the consumer. Dentists were enjoined to divest themselves from dental plans from which they directly benefited. The renamed Washington Dental Service was separated from the Washington State Dental Association in 1980. A similar progression occurred when the Oregon Dental Service and the California Dental Service were established in the same period. Employer-based dental benefits were now firmly entrenched within the commercial sector and opened access to dental care to a wider community for which dentists continued to thrive.

What is dental insurance?

One important way to improve America's oral health is to increase the number of individuals who have dental insurance because to have dental insurance drives individuals to seek dental care. Individuals with dental insurance are more than twice as likely to visit the dentist as those without insurance. Dental practices flourished when employer-based group dental plans became available during the 1960s.

There are a number of dental payment terms that are sometimes used interchangeably. Some of these terms are indemnity insurance, dental benefit plan, preferred provider organization (PPO), health maintenance organizations (HMO), direct service plan, direct reimbursement plan, discount plan, and administrative services only (ASO). Newer terms are ACO applied to Medicaid plans and CCO applied to commercial plans.

Indemnity insurance

Indemnity insurance can be thought of as pure insurance that reimburses for a loss. Members select any dentist for their care and the member is reimbursed on a fee-for-service basis up to a fixed amount. There is no relationship between the dentist and the insurer. Members are responsible for any differences between the insurance payment and the dentist's charge. In this arrangement, the dentist charges their retail fee, the usual, customary, and reasonable fee (UCR), which is based on what other providers in their geographic area charge for the same service.

The arrangement is between the insured and the insurer; think of automobile collision insurance. In this arrangement, the dentist charges their retail fee, the usual, customary, and reasonable fee (UCR), that is based on what providers in their geographic usually charge for the same service. The UCR in private practice is elastic where some patients are charged more and some charged less. The UCR in private practice is not derived from cost-based accounting but rather a what-the-market-will-bear strategy. The incentive for the provider's income control focuses on fee increases rather than expense decreases. Pure dental care indemnity insurance plans are rare. Those that seem to be dental insurance plans are merely dental benefit plans with liberal fee and utilization policy like the first dental benefit companies in the 1950s.

Dental benefit plan

Most group dental purchases are designed around dental benefit service plans. Dental benefit service plans are those in which the dentist and plan enter into a participating dentist agreement where certain activities between the dentist and the plan are codified. Dentists agree to be credentialed to become part of a panel of providers with access to a subscriber base. Fee allowances are negotiated in advance. The dental benefit plan can be designed as a fee-for-service plan or a capitation plan. Dental benefit service plans offer the purchasers of the dental benefits, usually employer groups or unions, a panel of dentists, quality oversight, utilization review, and financial risk mitigation.

The participating provider agreement is a binding contract between the dentist and the benefit company that delineates each party's responsibility to the member. There is no obligation for a dentist to participate and no obligation for a benefit plan to accept a dentist. One contractual issue is the most-favored-nation clause where the participating dentist agrees not to charge the subscriber any fee higher than a fee from another dental benefit plan, that is, the most favorable terms. The most-favored-nation clause is rarely invoked. Another issue is the noncovered service clause where the dentist agrees to limit their charge for a service to a predetermined amount for a service that is not covered by the dental plan. Thirty-three states have legislation that disallows noncovered service limitation (Table 1.1).

PPO

The PPO allows subscribers to receive dental care from a panel of participating dentists. The participating dentist agrees to abide by the provisions of the participating dentist agreement, submits claims on behalf of the plan member, and is directly reimbursed fee for service on predefined terms with a limitation on the maximum fee allowed. This type of benefit plan provides discounted fees and substantial savings to the subscriber, as long as the subscriber selects a dentist within the plan's network of participating providers. A nonparticipating dentist is usually reimbursed at a lower fee and the member is responsible to pay any balance the nonparticipating dentist chooses. In PPO plan subset design, the

Table 1.1 States with noncovered service legislation. https://wf.employeebenefitservice.com/
wps/wcm/connect/Storefronts/obc/1398878240638

State	Year	State	Year	State	Year
Alaska	2010	Kentucky	2012	Oklahoma	2010
Arkansas	2011	Louisiana	2011	Oregon	2010
Arizona	2011	Maryland	2011	Pennsylvania	2012
California	2011	Minnesota	2011	Rhode Island	2009
Connecticut	2012	Mississippi	2010	South Dakota	2010
Florida	2014	Missouri	2013	Tennessee	2011
Georgia	2011	Montana	2013	Texas	2011
Idaho	2010	Nebraska	2012	Virginia	2010
Illinois	2013	New Mexico	2011	Washington	2010
Iowa	2010	North Carolina	2010	Wisconsin	2014
Kansas	2010	North Dakota	2011	Wyoming	2011

Data from Ameritas 2010. © 2010, Wiley.

exclusive provider organization (EPO), all the PPO provisions apply except the member must select a PPO panel dentist to receive any dental benefit with a non-participating dentist not eligible for any reimbursement from the EPO plan.

HMO

A less common dental benefit plan design is the HMO that is sometimes called capitation or capitated plans. In this instance, the dentist or dental group is reimbursed for dental services on a per-member per-month basis rather than a fee-for-service rate. The capitated rate is a single fee paid per member per month to deliver all the dental care required of the member. For certain procedures, a copayment is allowed to be collected from the member. This plan design works when the member base is stable without adverse selection. A dentist participating in a HMO plan assumes financial risk for the set of patients.

In the best case where there is a sufficient patient base, all eligible HMO members are assigned to the dentists on the first day regardless of dental need, there is no adverse selection, and members remain with the dentist for the long term. These prerequisites for a successful HMO arrangement are rarely met in full. So to accept an HMO plan is risky for the dentist especially the solo dentist. HMO plans are more appropriate for dental groups. Most dental insurance companies offer an HMO product although a small part of their portfolio.

Direct service plan

The HMO resembles but is quite different from a direct service plan. The HMO finances dental care on a capitated basis and the dental services are delivered by other entities. Direct service plans both finances and delivers the dental care as a single entity. Western Dental (California) is both a dental direct service plan and a corporate dental entity. Western holds a California Knox-Keene license that allows it to sell HMO dental benefits, and Western also delivers dental care for its HMO products in its own offices in California and Arizona. Western Dental is a straightforward corporate entity enabled by its Knox-Keene license to operate its facilities and dental group without the convolutions required of other corporate entities. In some respects, it resembles a Kaiser Permanente model except it accepts patients other than its HMO policyholders.

While the direct service model showed promise to deliver health care to a wide range of people with a cost within a family's budget, the thought of a physician being employed by this system was anathema to organized medicine and the model was strongly resisted. Ross-Loos medical group in Los Angeles, California, and Sydney Garfield with Kaiser Permanente were the early adopters of this model. In dentistry, the model is less widely represented and usually relegated to specific population segment.

Direct reimbursement plan

A direct reimbursement plan is neither a dental insurance plan nor a dental benefit plan. It is a self-funded employer dental plan in which the employer reimburses the employee directly for all or part of their dental expenditures. Like an ASO plan, direct reimbursement plans are usually administered by a dental benefit company. In direct reimbursement, the employee chooses their dentist, pays the charge directly to the dentist, submits the receipt, and receives reimbursement. The reimbursement is usually based on a percent of the dollars expended for dental care and not for a specific procedure. There is an annual maximum.

A direct reimbursement plan does not moderate fees a dentist charges to the employee. There is no ceiling except what the traffic bears. The fee charged for a procedure can vary between dentists and can vary within the dental practice. Direct reimbursement is the design favored by dentists because of the freedom to charge the retail fee without oversight for the quality or quantity of services.

There are a number of reasons why direct reimbursement plans are an insignificant part of the dental benefit market in comparison to other benefit plan designs. The primary reason for microscopic market share and no growth, even with the support of organized dentistry, is that direct reimbursement plans are designed to benefit the dentist and not the subscriber or the payer. Carte blanche and rubber stamp plan designs overrely on the lack of moral hazard among providers and are inherently not consumer friendly.

Discount plan

Discount plans are neither insurance nor dental benefit. Rather, the discount plan is a fee list of discounted dental fees available to discount plan members. There may be a membership fee but there is no premium, waiting period, or exclusions. A dentist agrees to accept the discounted fee from plan members in exchange for the plans access to its members. Some dentists offer their own private label discount plan. To combine a discount plan in conjunction with a member's dental benefit plan may cause conflict with the dental plan's participating agreement.

For a discount plan to add certain prepaid benefit features like free diagnostic and preventive services may be in conflict with the state insurance law. The worst permutation of a discount plan is a percent discount on dental fees because the provider can change fees on a whim and the consumer rarely has access to fees in the community.

ASO

ASO can be thought of as a third-party administrator (TPA) that handles the administration of an employer self-funded dental plan. The administrative services offered include any or all of the benefit plan's services including actuarial analysis, plan design, claims processing, and the dental provider network.

The ASO plan and a dental benefit plan offered by the same benefit company will look the same to both the subscriber and the dentist. The eligibility, deductible, fee schedule, and Evidence of Coverage are identical.

The difference between ASO and a dental benefit plan is the employer (payer) in an ASO assumes all of the financial risk of utilization while the dental benefit company assumes the financial risk in a dental benefit plan.

For an ASO plan, the dental benefit company has little latitude to authorize payments outside of the plan design (it's not their money). In a dental benefit plan, the dental benefit company has wide latitude to authorize payments outside of the plan design (it's all their loss). For instance, when a subscriber is not reimbursed for services because a nonparticipating dentist treated them, there is no opportunity for a pay-and-teach in an ASO plan but pay-and-teach is frequently done in a dental benefit plan.

Bundled payment

In 2013, the Centers for Medicare & Medicaid Services introduced Bundled Payments for Care Improvement where organizations entered into payment arrangements that include financial and performance accountability for episodes of care. The episode of care methodology is an innovative initiative to replace the traditional fee-for-service payment for individual procedures or course of treatment that results in fragmented care with minimal coordination across providers and health-care settings. Fee-for-service rewards the quantity of services delivered rather than the quality or coordination of care. Episodes of dental care are currently bundled with medical care in the community health clinic setting.

Bundled payment and the episodes of care concept can be effectively introduced into the dental care setting with the adoption of dental diagnosis codes. For instance, bundled payment for a periodontal disease episode of care would be identified with a diagnostic code and ultimately reward the nonrecurrence of periodontal disease. The bundled payment system is the interim step away from fee-for-service payment for the quantity of service and toward an integrated system like the accountable care or coordinated care system that rewards health outcome and disease management.

ACO

An ACO is a group of hospitals, physicians, and affiliated health-care providers who gather under an umbrella organization to deliver coordinated care to a population. Payment is through some form of bundled payment. The goal is to give the right care, at the right time, in the right amount and avoid duplication of services. The ACO shares in the savings it achieves through cost-efficient care.

The Centers for Medicare & Medicaid Services introduced the ACO model for its Medicare members. Oregon developed its CCO model built around the Triple Aim. Oregon implemented its Medicaid program by dividing the state into regions with one CCO designated to care for Medicare members in each region. Oregon's CCOs will next extend their services to state employees and other health-care payers through strategies that emphasize alternative payment models, patient-centered primary care, and robust quality measures for accountability. Oregon's vision is to create a health system in which oral health is integrated and coordinated.

It's reported that one Silicon Valley technology company moved from its health insurer and their provider network to a physician-controlled ACO to provide health care for its employees. The ACO concept is moving from serving federal programs to the private sector. Dentists and dental practice will be impacted when ACOs in the private sector integrate dental care as an important component of overall health care.

Antitrust

Dentists feel that there is unfair weight of the law when they deal with the third-party payers of dental benefits. Insurance companies enjoy financial heft and reach that surpass any individual dentist. It seems only fair that individual small practice owners in a community can band together in a show of force to present a countervailing force to insurance companies and negotiate favorable terms with the third-party payers. But as you know, this is per se illegal and a violation of the Sherman Antitrust Act. A per se violation is inherently illegal and requires no further inquiry into the actual effect on the market or the intentions of the individuals. For individual dentists to conspire to lower fees is equally per se illegal and a prohibited action. To individual dentists, there appears to be a disparity in the bargaining power between providers and payers, but the government does not believe that monopsony power exists in most health-care markets.

Even if it were assumed that providers confront monopsony health plans, the government believes that to allow providers to exercise countervailing power doesn't serve the consumers' interests. This is not a trivial issue for individual dentists. In *United States v. A. Lanoy Alston et al.*, the defendants were convicted in a criminal case for a concerted action to conspire to fix and raise their copayment fee (Box 1.1).

Box 1.1 Antitrust

United States v. A. Lanoy Alston et al.
The case was the first criminal case the Antitrust Division brought against medical practitioners in over 50 years. The Justice Department charged three dentists with conspiracy to fix and raise the copayment fees paid to the dentists from four prepaid dental plans in the Tucson area. In Tucson, some dentists failed to break even on some common services like porcelain crowns. Several Tucson dentists individually requested fee increases but were rejected. Subsequently, 50 local dentists met to discuss the copayment fees from prepaid dental health plans, which had not risen for 10 years and were lower than fees in Phoenix. The government contended that the defendants agreed to persuade the health plans to raise their copayments and then mailed identical letters demanding a higher fee schedule. The Justice Department contended the dentists met with the intention to exert pressure on the plans to raise fees. The dentists claimed they met, *at the behest of president of one of the plans*, to justify, in a show of show-of-force, a new copayment schedule that would rationalize fees between Tucson and Phoenix. The Justice Department alleged that the conspiracy caused the dental plans to pay higher copayment fees than they might otherwise had to pay. The case was tried in December 1990, and the jury found all the three defendants guilty. In January 1993, the Government reached a settlement with all parties.

Conclusion

Dentists practicing today have always worked in a world of dental benefits. It is a way of life that has remained essentially unchanged since the inception of the dental benefit service company in the 1950s. Dental insurance is a benefit of employment with the employee having very little input to a plan design. Dental care is delivered through small private practice and the dentist is paid fee for service. The dentist considers the provider–patient relationship sacrosanct with third-party scrutiny detrimental to quality of care. The dentist is accountable to only their patient.

Given a shifting payment environment, it is incumbent upon each dentist to understand how dental benefits work and how they can efficiently manage the current and emerging systems of dental care payment. The rising cost of health-care services as percent of GDP is rising and is not sustainable. The emerging models of payment for services and dental care delivery attempt to control the cost of care while extending access to care to more individuals. Patient-centered care and a streamlined office process are key elements to the emerging models.

As dental benefits become uncoupled from employment, the fee-for-service method of payment is being evaluated for sustainability, procedures are being linked to diagnosis, more individuals have access dental care, and payers look to cost-effective care with positive health outcomes.

So, to understand the history of the prepayment of health-care services and the future vision of dental care delivery is the essential first step for a dentist to design a sustainable and competitive model of care for the future. This chapter describes the past and present states of dental care payment and the tentative forays into the future state of dental care payment through ACO and bundled payment. Dentists just entering into dental practice can look back at what was successful for their colleagues but shouldn't rely on past successes to model their future behavior and strategy for success.

Further reading

Marmor TR. *The Politics of Medicare*. Aldine Publishing Company: Chicago, 1973.
Schoen MH. *Observation of Selected Dental Services Under Two Prepayment Mechanisms (DrPH Dissertation)*. University of California, Los Angeles, 1969.
Starr P. *The Social Transformation of American Medicine*. Basic Books: New York, 1982.

CHAPTER 2

Dental benefits: Get it done

Michael M. Okuji

Delta Dental of Colorado, Denver, USA

Introduction

To understand the dental claim form and the Code on Dental Procedures and Nomenclature (CDT code) is essential to the business of dentistry. To fully understand these processes is something not to be delegated. They are not obstacles to dental care but underpin the documentation of treatment.

This chapter is designed to assist you to understand how to efficiently and accurately submit dental claims for the payment of services. The universal claim form and the CDT code set are the bedrock to do this. The CDT code is the important language because the clinical data that is collected at each patient encounter populates both the clinical record and the dental claim form. The CDT code is the lingua franca by which everyone in dental reimbursement system, provider–administrator–third-party payer, must use to understand one another. Mastering this arcane language enables the effective and efficient administrative process that must be built into everyday practice.

Mastering procedure codes and dental claim submission is important for two reasons. Firstly, the CDT code is the federal government Health Insurance Portability and Accountability Act (HIPAA) standard for reporting dental procedures on dental claims and is the default code for dental treatment recording. Secondly, it is likely that a dental benefit pays for some portion of the cost of care, so accurate submission of a dental claim is a prerequisite to payment. Today, 60% of the population has some form of dental benefit through their employer. Other groups with dental benefits include public programs like Medicaid, Child Health Plan Plus (CHP+), and the military Tricare program that provides dental coverage through civilian care. Almost all dental benefits are provided through an employer or other group coverages. Very little is purchased by individuals. This, in itself, is a compelling reason to master insurance submission procedures.

The mix between group and individual purchasing behavior is likely to drastically change as more consumers begin to purchase dental benefits on the public

Dental Benefits and Practice Management: A Guide for Successful Practices, First Edition.
Edited by Michael M. Okuji.
© 2016 John Wiley & Sons, Inc. Published 2016 by John Wiley & Sons, Inc.

exchange through provisions of the Affordable Care Act and employers shift employee dental benefits to off-exchange purchases.

To understand the engine that runs your practice is of paramount importance for clear recording on the clinical record and smooth administration of the financial record. This chapter steps into the shoes of the front office staff and dental benefit administrator to understand the features of the universal claim form and the CDT code.

Dental benefits

As we saw in Chapter 1, "Why Dental Benefits," the individual purchaser of a health-care service has long sought to modulate the cost of care through group purchasing power. Purchasing groups started as fraternal groups and immigrant societies on the East Coast and expanded to employer delivered care in the railroad and mining industries. The further expansion of purchasing health-care services through third parties expanded the number of stakeholders beyond just the provider and patient.

Stakeholders in the financing of dental care comprise a number of layers that include the patient, provider, employer, regulator, and dental plan. Each plays a role to balance the interests of the other.

Patients, as consumers, seek to mitigate the cost of an unforeseen, catastrophic health. Dental care rarely falls into this category of health service. Dental benefits are designed to provide financial assistance for health events that are high in frequency but relatively low cost and predictable. Consumers with a dental benefit are more than twice as likely to visit the dentist.

It's further seen that there exists a considerable difference between dental conditions and their reimbursement from medical conditions and their reimbursement (Table 2.1). Everyday dental care is principally limited to just two conditions, dental caries and periodontal disease. Dental conditions are predicable and understood by the patient and are of high frequency with relatively low cost. In contrast, medical conditions are widely diverse, not predictable, infrequent in occurrence, and with cost fluctuation that can be catastrophic.

Employers are the primary source of dental benefits. Individual dental benefit plans are rarely purchased. Dental benefits are an important employee benefit

Table 2.1 Dental versus medical insurance.

Dental benefit	Medical insurance
Caries and periodontal disease	Wide range of medical conditions
Predictable and costless variable	Not predictable and cost can fluctuate
High frequency—low cost	Infrequent—catastrophic cost

and competitive advantage for employers to hire and retain their workforce. Employers negotiate for low premiums, access to providers, and cost savings for their employees. However, employers are faced with increasing health-care costs and seek ways to control that cost through increased employee contributions, maintain benefits and move to 100% voluntary employee paid, and move employees to off-exchange purchases. This impacts the policy and payment for dental care services through dental benefit plans.

Regulators play a role to assure that the consumer interests are put at the forefront of accurate, timely, and transparent payment of benefits. Prepaid dental benefits are under the purview of regulators. This can extend to certain dental plans offered by individual dental offices that proffer discount plans with monthly service fees and no-charge service. A state's Department of Insurance of the Department of Managed Health Care (California) has oversight for prepaid dental plans with a number of enforceable consumer protection functions.

Dentists are acutely aware that the existence of a dental benefit increases the likelihood that a consumer will seek dental services. Participation in a dental plan network enables the dentist to engage a wider audience of potential patients than they would otherwise engage. The opportunity to grow a practice is higher with participation than without.

The existence of dental benefits introduces the dentist, patient, employer, state regulator, and third-party payer into the dental benefit mix. Each party benefits and is better off from the others participating.

Plan design

Dental benefit plans purchased by employers are of two types. First is the risk plan. Second is the administrative services only (ASO). Each carries different sets of operating processes that aren't readily understood by the patient and the provider.

Risk plans are those in which the dental plan company assumes the financial risk of utilization. Since the benefit company assumes financial risk, any change to the scope and/or breadth of the procedure payment is more readily actuated. For instance, if a misunderstanding by the provider or patient on the claim results in nonpayment, the benefit company may allow payment as a pay-and-educate opportunity. This can happen when a compliant dental plan under the Affordable Care Act requires payment to only a participating dentist and the patient seeks care from a nonparticipating dentist.

ASO plans are those in which the dental plan company administers the provider network and administration of payment, but the financial risk of utilization is borne by the employer, the purchaser. These are also called self-insured plan. In this case, a pay-and-educate opportunity is under the purview of the employer, not the benefit company.

The Employee Retirement Income Security Act (ERISA) plans are those that are governed under the federal law—not the state law. ERISA plans are typically self-funded through large employers, associations, union, and government entities.

Participating provider agreement

The singular feature that sets dental benefits apart from dental insurance is the participating provider agreement. In this world, a dentist is either participating or nonparticipating provider depending on whether they are contracted or noncontracted. When the employer that purchases their dental benefit, whether a risk plan or an ASO plan, through a dental benefit company, they also purchase access to the benefit company's provider network. Dentists that choose to participate in a network execute a participating provider agreement. This is a contractual agreement between the dentist and the dental benefit company that affirms the terms in which the dentist agrees to submit claims for payment. These terms vary from company to company. It is important that each agreement is read and understood, as cringeworthy as it is to do. No two agreements are entirely the same. Participating provider agreements are binding contracts.

Features of a participating provider agreement revolve around fees, billing policy, submitted fee, allowed fee, paid amount formula, covered service, frequency, adjudication, and the appeal process. There are features on the timely filing, predetermination of services, assignment of benefit, and coordination of benefit. Exclusions and limitations are specific to an individual policy. Agreements may refer to dentally necessary or dental necessity that means a service that a dentist exercising prudent clinical judgment would provide. Agreements may refer to least expensive alternative treatment (LEAT) when there are multiple options that lead to the same outcome.

The participating provider agreement is a business relationship between the dentist and the third-party payer. The agreement delineates the responsibility and benefit of the business relationship including the terms and termination of the relationship.

There is the notion of being in network (participating) and out of network (nonparticipating) that may affect the amount of reimbursement and the patient's ultimate out-of-pocket expense. In some cases, the patient who seeks an out of network for care may be reimbursed at a lower rate or maybe not at all.

There is the notion of participating in a leased network. In this case, a dentist signs a participating dentist agreement with one benefit company that subsequently leases the dentist's contract to another company. The dentist then begins to receive explanation of benefit (EOB) reports from a benefit company that the dentist never engaged.

Credentialing

After executing the participating provider agreement, the benefit company reviews the credentials of the provider. Each company has its own credential application form with required supporting documentation. Some states mandate a common credentialing application form for all health-care professionals in that state that ask questions not applicable to most dentists. Commonly requested supporting documents are dental license, evidence of liability insurance, Basic Life Support certificate, and Drug Enforcement Agency number. Benefit companies routinely scan the state dental board and the National Practitioner Data Bank websites for reported actions. Be prepared to truthfully respond to any reports from these sources. Dentists are initially credentialed and then recredentialed every 3–4 years to remain eligible to participate in the provider network. Credentialing is established to assure that each participating dentist meets certain standards for licensure, certification, and liability insurance coverage. Some companies adopt the National Committee for Quality Assurance (NCQA) guidelines or the Utilization Review Accreditation Commission (URAC) guidelines.

Medicare opt-in/opt-out

The Centers for Medicare and Medicaid Services (CMS) requires dentists who treat or refer Medicare enrollees or prescribe medication to Medicare patients through Part D of the Medicare program to designate their status as a Medicare provider. There are three options available for the dentist to comply with this regulation: opt-in, opt-out, or an ordering and referring provider.

Opt-in option allows a dentist that delivers Medicare-covered services to a Medicare enrollee to be reimbursed by Medicare. Medicare covers certain dental procedures that have a corresponding medical code like oral surgery, periodontal surgery, laboratory order, and prescriptions. Dental practices that serve a senior population will benefit from the opt-in option.

Opt-out option alerts the CMS that the dentist chooses not to participate in Medicare. Any senior that participates in Medicare and is seen by a dentist that elects to opt out of Medicare must enter into a written private contract with the dentist (Box 2.1). The contract specifies that payment of dental services must be paid in full by the patient. The dentist will not submit, nor can the patient submit on their own behalf, a dental claim for dental service to Medicare. The opt-out

Box 2.1 Medicare Private Contract: Sample

I understand that Michael Okuji, DDS, has opted out of the Medicare program.

I understand that no claims will be submitted to Medicare for services and no Medicare reimbursement will be provided for these services. I understand and agree that I will not submit or request Michael Okuji, DDS, to submit a claim to Medicare or its agents for services provided by him even if such services are otherwise covered.

I understand that a Medigap plan does not and other health and medical care insurance plans, like a Medicare Advantage plan, may not make payments for services rendered by me.

I agree to be fully responsible to pay for services rendered by Michael Okuji, DDS. I understand that there is no limit specified by Medicare as to the amounts that I can charge you for the dental services that I provide.

I further understand that I have the right to have dental services provided by another dentist who elects to opt in to Medicare and for whom a Medicare payment may be made.

Reproduced with permission from Kristopher Hart. © Kristopher Hart, Medicare Private Care.

dentist cannot submit a claim even if the procedure is a covered Medicare benefit. The opt-out is an active process in which the dentist must submit an affidavit attesting to their opt-out status to the Medicare administrator for the region. The opt-out status must be renewed every 2 years.

The ordering and referring provider option enrollment places the dentist in the Medicare system. This option does not allow the dentist to bill Medicare for their services but does allow the referral of a Medicare enrollee to another opt-in dentist or a pharmacist to fill their prescriptions or laboratory for tests.

If a dentist elects to neither opt in, opt out, nor become an ordering and referring provider because their expectation is to never provide a Medicare-covered service or never refer for a Medicare-covered service, they can do nothing. The negative ramification of the do-nothing decision travels downstream when a Medicare provider, like a laboratory or pharmacy, is referred a patient by a do-nothing dentist and is not reimbursed for their service by Medicare. If the patient of a do-nothing dentist submits a claim on their own behalf, Medicare will notify the patient that the dentist needs to enroll in the Medicare system.

Fees

The crux of tension between the patient, dentist, and the benefit company is often fees. One aspect of fees is what fee for a procedure is allowed for computation of the benefit. In some cases, it's the filed fee method in which a dentist submits their office fee schedule and the benefit company either accepts or rejects or recomputes the fee schedule. In other cases, it's the fee schedule methodology in which the dental benefit company lists a fee schedule and the dentist either accepts it to become a participating provider or rejects it and becomes a nonparticipating provider (Table 2.2).

A dental benefit company may choose to negotiate a set of fees with the provider. This is the case if a provider practices in a strategic location or the benefit company wants to build a bigger network in the region. To negotiate a higher fee doesn't guarantee that any patient will seek services.

Table 2.2 Benefit plan fee definitions.

Term	Definition
Submitted fee	The fee charged to a patient regardless of benefit coverage
Allowed fee	The maximum fee chargeable to the patient
Paid fee	The benefit computed from the allowed fee
Patient portion	The difference between the allowed and paid fee
Deny	No benefit and the service chargeable to the patient up to the allowed amount
Disallow	No benefit and the service is not chargeable to the patient

Dental claim form (American Dental Association)

The American Dental Association (ADA) dental claim form is the national format recognized by third-party payers, including federal programs, to submit dental claims for service either electronically or by paper. The ADA claim form is HIPAA compliant. Always use the most current format because fields are changed, added, and deleted. Form J430D was issued in 2012 and certain fields to review are highlighted.

It is critically important for the dental office to fully and accurately submit a claim to assure that all procedures are accounted. An incomplete or inaccurate claim results in requests for additional information that delays processing or a denied payment because the description doesn't capture the essence of the procedure.

The nature of a prepayment system and benefit payment requires documentation and a vehicle for submission of services. This requires the dentist to understand both the claim system (ADA dental claim form) and the language of procedures (CDT code) in order to submit a claim through the ofttime onerous process. To understand the system and develop administrative systems takes a considerable amount of time and is something a dentist delegates at their peril.

While some providers feel that it's the patient's responsibility to understand their dental benefit plan and they bear the responsibility for its adjudication, other providers feel that it's just another part of operating a successful dental business; smooth and efficient claim processes are good for the patient and good for the dentist. After all, how many dentists understand their medical policy and the cost for a broken arm?

Dental claim field changes (2012)

Most of the 58 separate fields in the ADA dental claim are automatically populated from the electronic dental record. The electronic information linkage eliminates repetitive rekeying between the operatory, front desk, and billing department.

Of the 58 available fields on the dental claim, five fields are of particular interest (Table 2.3). Mistakes here will delay claim adjudication or leads to misinformation:

Box 1, Header Information, contains the request for a predetermination or preauthorization. If this box is ticked, do not enter the date of service.

Table 2.3 Fields: Changed (2012).

Field	Name	Description
Box 1	Header Information	Predetermination or actual service
Box 3	Benefit Plan Information	Primary carrier address
Box 35	Remarks	Free form field
Box 36	Authorization	Financial responsibility
Box 53	Treating Dentist	Treating versus billing entity

This predetermination or preauthorization feature is underutilized. For an office to guesstimate more often than not leads to patient confusion and dissatisfaction when the office estimate differs even slightly from the actual benefit. The rule of thumb is to submit a case for predetermination if the provider would be distressed to adjust off a patient balance because of a misunderstanding. In many cases, a predetermination is returned in a matter of days when submitted electronically.

Box 3, Dental Benefit Plan Information, is where the dental benefit company address is entered for the initial submission of the claim. Be alert that some benefit companies have different billing addresses for related companies or separate subsidiaries, that is, a benefit company may have different plans with different billing addresses. To send the claim to the right company at the wrong address needlessly delays claim payment. Check the patient's insurance card for the correct billing address.

Box 35, Remarks, is where free form comments are entered. For a secondary claim, this is where to place the payment from the primary benefit plan. Remarks may kick the claim from an automatic adjudication queue (computer) to a reviewer queue (a person).

Box 36, Authorization, is for the patient's signature that recognizes that both the patient and the provider may have a contractual relationship with the same benefit company. The patient acknowledges that they are responsible for all fees not paid by their dental plan except if the provider has a contractual relationship with the same benefit company that prohibits a portion or all of the charge for service to the patient. It is disingenuous for a provider to say that a dental plan agreement is just between the patient and the plan when the provider has a separate agreement with the same benefit company. In this case, it is untrue for the provider to say they don't participate in the plan, and all fees are to be paid regardless of the benefit.

Box 53, Treating Dentist, is where the treating dentist certifies that treatment is in progress for procedures that require multiple visits or the treatment has been completed. Note that some provider agreements stipulate that procedures that require multiple visits are billed on the date of completion. As the number of employed dentists increases, it is common for the treating dentist to be different from the billing entity. For the treating dentist who is an employee, it is prudent to verify that the procedures attributed to them by the billing entity are correct. In the case of inaccurate billing, the treating dentist who is the employee is placed in the position of fraudulent billing of services. It is never appropriate to submit a claim with the treating dentist and the billing dentist as the same entity when it is not so.

Dental claim new fields

Eleven new fields were added to the 2012 version of the ADA dental claim (Table 2.4). These fields are added in anticipation of emerging trends in the reporting dental treatment, most notably diagnostic code. The box for "Other Fees" anticipates mandatory fees, like a sales tax, that may be imposed by regulatory agencies including the Affordable Care Act.

Table 2.4 Fields—new.

Field	Name	Description
Box 4	Other dental–medical coverages	Without regard to whether the dentist or patient will submit for payment
Box 15	Policyholder identifier	Unique identifying number assigned by insurer
Box 19	Reserved for future use	Leave blank
Box 29a	Diagnostic code pointer	Enter letter(s) from 34 that identify the diagnosis code(s) applicable to the dental procedure
Box 29b	Quantity	Number of times the procedure is delivered on the date of service in item 34
Box 31a	Other fees	Charges may include state tax and other regulatory fees
Box 33	Missing teeth information	"X" missing permanent teeth only when pertinent to the case
Box 34	Diagnostic code list qualifier	B = ICD-9-CM, AB = ICD-10-CM
Box 34a	Diagnosis code(s)	Up to 4 diagnostic codes per procedure
Box 38	Place of treatment	11 = office, 12 = home, 21 = inpatient, 22 = outpatient, 31 = skilled nursing home, 32 = nursing facility
Box 39	Number of enclosures (00–99)	Yes or no enclosures of any type

Box 4 changes how dental and medical coverage is entered when the patient has additional coverage. It is to be completed regardless of whether the provider or the patient will ever submit to the additional dental or medical entity for the payment of benefits.

Box 15 is to enter the policyholder's unique identifying number assigned by the employer or benefit company. For the sake of security, employers are moving away from using the Social Security number as the patient identifier to a unique employer assigned number. The patient cannot be matched to their dental plan when a dental office omits the unique identifying number.

Boxes 29a, 20b, and 34a recognize the emergence of the diagnosis codes in addition to the CDT procedure code. Box 34, Diagnostic Code List Qualifier, is important when the diagnosis code has impact on adjudication where the procedure minimizes the risk associated with oral and systemic health. The 2012 form supports up to four diagnostic codes per dental procedure. A diagnostic code set adds a layer of data that enables the tracking of efficacious treatment and outcome.

Box 31a is for other charges applicable to dental services. These charges may include state taxes and other charges imposed by regulatory agencies. While not common today, the future may hold a sales tax imposed on a dental service or dental device. New Mexico, Hawaii, and Minnesota have a sales tax on dental services. This field is not to report unspecified services like a convenience fee for the use of a special dental device. A convenience fee is more appropriately entered in the procedure code field with the appropriate CDT code, usually a Dx999.

Box 32 totals the procedure codes plus other charges in Box 31a.

Box 38 allows a 2-digit place of treatment field that's a HIPAA standard maintained by the CMS. Box 38 becomes significant to complete as dental treatment begins to be disbursed to nontraditional settings. Common 2-digit codes for Box 38 are 11—office, 12—home, 21—inpatient hospital, 22—outpatient hospital, 31—skilled nursing facility, and 32—nursing facility.

Box 39 allows for a yes or no to designate whether there are any number enclosures of any type included with the dental claim (like radiographs, photographs, periodontal chart, and narrative). This pertains to both paper and electronic claims.

National provider identification

Boxes 49 and 54 allow the national provider identification (NPI) for the billing entity and the treating dentist. The NPI number is a unique, government-issued identification number that dentists are required to obtain and use when they bill a claim electronically, use a clearinghouse to process a claim, use the Internet to verify patient eligibility, use the Internet to verify dental benefits, and use the Internet to check the status of a submitted claim. There are two types of NPI: Type 1 for the individual dentist and Type 2 for incorporated group practices. This means every dentist practicing in the 21st century should have an NPI number or is practicing off the grid. The dentist is responsible to update any change of information to the National Plan and Provider Enumeration System (NPPES) within 30 days of that change.

Tax identification number

Box 51 allows the tax identification number (TIN) or the dentist's Social Security number that is the identification number used by the Internal Revenue Service. Most businesses use the TIN. Some solo practitioners prefer to use their Social Security number.

Narrative attachment

Submission of a dental claim using the CDT code may not fully explain the circumstances leading to the procedure or to support a deviation from standard treatment. To establish clarity is where a narrative is useful. What is clear to the clinician may not be as clear to a reviewer.

Periodontal root plane and scale is indicated for patients with periodontal disease and is therapeutic and not prophylactic in nature. Hence, there is a requirement to demonstrate the presence of disease. Sometimes, pocket depths alone don't sufficiently illustrate bone loss. Additional information like furcation involvement, mobility, recession, and attached gingival loss may support the diagnosis and the need for the procedure. The reason to complete four quadrants in a single visit should be compelling and not just for the convenience of the patient or the dentist.

Full coverage in the instance of cracked tooth syndrome should be supported with the appropriate signs and symptoms. If the crack is not visible on a radiographic, is it visible clinically and documented in a photographic image? Were other diagnoses ruled out and was there consideration of palliative treatment prior to definitive treatment?

Customization of a crown should be documented as to need and supported by a photograph and/or a detailed laboratory order. Discolored teeth due tetracycline stain, fluorosis, and congenital enamel dysplasia are difficult to replicate and take a significant amount of time and talent to duplicate. This is easy to support as customization in a narrative. Normal porcelain layering, staining, and contouring are less easy to support as customization in a narrative.

Box 35, "Remarks," can be used if the narrative is indicated for a procedure and the remark is brief. Otherwise, reference in the Remarks section that a narrative is contained on a NEA attachment.

Needless to say, the objective of the narrative is to provide clarity. Don't assume that what you see or think is obvious to another dentist. Explain your point of view respectfully. This is not a platform to display superior knowledge in a condescending tone. Being passive aggressive doesn't work. You're trying to convince not the needle. In the end, consider other points of view and, within this framework of understanding, propose a solution. If you prevail, a sincere thank you; if you fail, don't sulk and threaten.

In addition to the narrative, other attachments to the dental claim are indicated for a number of procedures to support payment of a dental claim. A full periodontal chart with radiographs is often a required attachment for definitive therapeutic periodontal treatment. Attachments for a complex restorative treatment plan may include radiographs, photos of the dentition and preoperative study cast, preliminary workup, and laboratory order, along with the narrative.

Certain common customs are taken into consideration whenever a dental claim is submitted and a dental code entered (Table 2.5).

Code for what you do and not for what you think will be allowed. To do otherwise misleads the patient and the benefit company. To code this way has a tendency to leave a murky trail of the treatment that was actually rendered. This situation is the antithesis of what the clinical record aspires to be. The clinical record and the subsequent claim generated strive for clarity of thought and action to future readers of the dental record.

Enter all procedures performed without regard to whether they will be paid. To omit a code on a claim merely because it isn't covered or paid misconstrues the

Table 2.5 Claim filing hints.

Claim hints
Code for what is actually done and not for what might be allowed
Enter all procedures performed without regard to whether they will be paid
Enter the office's fee, not the fee that is allowed
Enter coinsurance coverage without regard to whether it will be submitted for payment

treatment rendered. The procedure code travels from the clinical record to the dental claim and gives the only clear evidence of what actually was performed. It is of importance that the treating dentist records all the actual treatment rendered so the patient and any future treating clinician correctly understand the treatment flow. Epidemiologic evaluation is impossible without a complete dental record as reported on a dental claim.

Enter the office's actual fee for the procedure, not the fee that will be allowed. This is the most accurate way to monitor and evaluate the fees actually charged in the office. To do otherwise results in mishmash of fees for a single procedure that makes meaningful financial analysis impossible.

Enter all coinsurance coverage without regard to whether the dentist or patient will submit it for payment. Coinsurance is the case where an individual is covered by two policies at the same time. This can be the individual's policy and the spouse's policy or the child covered by both parents' policy. This information may increase the breadth and/or depth of coverage or contribute to the data incorporated in insurance rate setting policy. Completing this section accurately ultimately benefits both the dentist and the patient.

EOB

The EOB is a written statement sent to the patient and the provider that explains how the claim was adjudicated (Table 2.6). The EOB typically shows the submitted fee, allowed fee, deductible applied, coinsurance percent, patient pay amount, and plan pay amount. There is also a Remarks field with an identifier or delimiter. The Remarks field pertains to the adjudication of the benefit and explains how the benefit is computed. Remarks are never meant to guide a treatment decision that is under the purview of the patient and the provider. Nor do Remarks imply that the provider utilized a wrong procedure code or has inappropriate submitted fees. If the wording of the Remark seems to imply anything but an adjudication computation, the provider can request the benefit company to change its EOB language. The electronic version of the EOB is the electronic remittance advice (ERA).

Financial information like the EOB should be separate from the dental record. Other financial records that are not part of the dental record are financial ledger card, insurance claims, and payment reconciliation report.

CDT code

The CDT code, sometimes referred to as Current Dental Terminology, is the reference manual for dental procedures. The CDT code's principle use is to provide a uniform, consistent, and specific means to transmit procedure information in a dental claim. It is useful as a common professional language for dental professionals and educational institutions. The CDT code has become the default language for treatment planing and the clinical dental record.

Table 2.6 Explanation of benefit (EOB) fields.

Service date	Description of service	Procedure code	Tooth number	Submitted fee	Allowed fee	Deductible	%	Patient pays	Plan pays	Remark
1/1/2xxx	Evaluation	D0xxx	–	$44	$44	$00	100%	$00	$44	–
1/1/2xxx	Prophylaxis	D1xxx	–	$83	$83	$00	100%	$00	$83	–
1/1/2xxx	Amalgam	D2xxx	3	$125	$116	$50	80%	$63.20	$52.80	777

Plan pay $179.80

Patient pay $63.20

Remarks 777 fee exceeds plan allowance.

If the ADA dental claim form is the book, the CDT code is language. The provider stands in good stead when they become bilingual and fluent in the language of dentistry.

The CDT code is maintained and published annually by the ADA. The CDT code was first published in 1969 as the "Uniform Code on Dental Procedures and Nomenclature" in the *Journal of the American Dental Association.* Since 1990, the ADA has published the CDT code in a reference manual called "Current Dental Terminology" that first contained a descriptor (narrative) in addition to the number and nomenclature (title). The CDT code and the CDT reference manual are the intellectual property of the ADA, which owns the copyright. The CDT code is the named HIPAA national standard to document dental procedures to submit to third-party payers electronically. Dental practice management software utilizes the CDT code to populate the office dental record.

> The existence of a specific CDT code does not guarantee that the procedure is a covered dental benefit that must be paid by a third-party payer.

CDT code use

The CDT code categorizes and describes the procedure performed—what was done. The CDT code doesn't separately categorize, for claim submission purposes, the tool used, for example, laser, or a specific protocol, for example, laser-assisted new attachment procedure.

The CDT code doesn't recognize unbundling of procedures to its component parts in order for each component to be billed separately. For instance, components of a full coverage crown include the preparation, impression, temporization, fabrication, and seat of the crown. Normal steps in the preparation include anesthesia, preparation of the tooth, tissue management, impression tray, impression, and temporary crown. Normal parts of the crown fabrication include the working model, material used, contouring, establishing occlusion, porcelain stacking or milling, staining, and the glaze. So to break out anesthesia, temporization, and ceramic customization as a separate charge is to submit them as a Dx999, unspecified by report code, and reviewed and adjudicated on the merits. The same is true of periodontal scaling and root planing when a separate gross debridement or prophylaxis procedure performed on the same day of service is submitted for payment. Is gross debridement or prophylaxis a fundamental part of the underlying root planing procedure?

Every CDT code procedure is composed of at least two of three parts (Figure 2.1). The first part is the procedure code, a five-character alphanumeric code that begins with the letter "D" followed by four numbers. The letter "D" denotes dental. The second part is nomenclature that is the title of the procedure code. The third part is the descriptor that is a narrative that further defines and describes the intended use of the particular procedure code. All procedures contain a procedure code number and a descriptor. Not all procedures contain a descriptor.

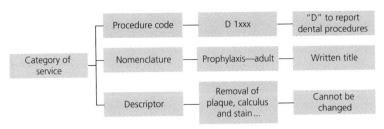

Figure 2.1 CDT code description.

Descriptors that apply to series of procedure codes precede the series of codes. For instance, in addition to their individual descriptors, the clinical oral evaluation code subcategory begins by recognizing the cognitive skills necessary for patient evaluation that is beyond the ken of nondentist providers. Nondentist provider evaluation codes are contained in the prediagnostic service subcategory.

The CDT code set seeks clarity for claim submission and communication and data aggregation. To meet the test, definitions and rules are written that satisfy the needs of the clinician in most instances. However, not everything fits into a neat bucket for the everyday practice of dentistry. For this, it requires a studied approach to mastering the code. The following are examples of situations that don't fit neatly within the code.

An amalgam filling has a procedure code in the D21xx range with nomenclature, amalgam—one surface, primary or permanent teeth, and no descriptor. Pediatric dentists may balk at nomenclature that lumps primary and permanent amalgams under one procedure code.

A single full coverage crown on a natural tooth has a procedure code in the D27xx range with nomenclature, crown—porcelain fused to metal, and no descriptor. Nowhere in the nomenclature does it mention a freestanding single crown on a natural tooth. The experienced clinician understands that a different procedure code applies to a single crown on a natural tooth that is an abutment for a fixed partial denture (D67xx) or a single crown on an abutment above an implant body (D60xx).

A prophylaxis—child D1xxx is for the removal of plaque, calculus, and stains from the tooth structures in the primary and transitional dentition. It is intended to control local factors that cause gingival irritation. This code is age banded and applied to the age of the patient regardless of the development of the permanent teeth. For instance, if a dental plan defines a child as up to age 15 and the child has all their permanent teeth at age 14, the appropriate code is prophylaxis—child (not prophylaxis—adult), even in the presence of all their succedaneous teeth. Also, the time required for a prophylaxis—child on a 5-year-old with plaque versus a 15-year-old with calculus doesn't change the prophylaxis code.

Periodontal scaling and root planing is a definitive therapeutic procedure in the presence of disease. It is not a replacement code for a difficult prophylaxis. To plane a root surface requires the root surface to be exposed. There must be some bone loss. The presence of pseudopocket alone does not alone justify periodontal scaling and root planing. An attached periodontal chart and a notation in Box 35, "Remarks," are suggested to support the procedure and document the need.

Dx999, "Unspecified diagnostic procedure, by report," is the last CDT code in each category section. It is used for procedures that aren't adequately described by any code in that category. A written report is required for this code. A written report describing the procedure can be entered in Box 35, "Remarks," or on a separate narrative attachment. Box 35 of the dental claim and the narrative reflects the entry in the dental record and never replaces the dental record.

These nuances of the CDT code language are easily learned because most dentists practice in a world of limited number of procedure codes—perhaps 50—and soon become fluent and understand the idiosyncrasies of the dental procedure language.

Categories of service

The CDT code procedure set is organized into twelve categories of service (Figure 2.2). A category can be organized into a subcategory and a subdivision of related procedures. Categorization promotes ease of understanding since dentists practice within a limited set of procedure codes and can focus their learning on those categories they use in everyday practice. A restorative general dentist uses at least six categories, I, II, III, VI, VIII, and IX. An endodontist lives in category IV.

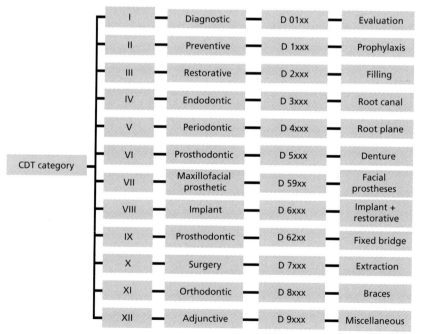

Figure 2.2 CDT code category.

Table 2.7 Category subdivision.

Category VIII	Implant services
Subcategory	Implant-supported prosthetics
Subdivision	Supporting structure
	Implant-/abutment-supported removable denture
	Implant-/abutment-supported fixed denture
	Single crown, abutment supported
	Single crown, implant supported
	Fixed partial denture, abutment supported
	Fixed partial denture, implant supported

Table 2.8 Single crown codes.

Procedure	Tooth replaced	Restoration	CDT series
Single crown	Natural tooth	Single tooth	D27XX
Single crown	Natural tooth	Abutment fixed partial denture	D67XX
Single crown	Implant support abutment	Single tooth	D60XX
Single crown	Implant support abutment	Abutment fixed partial denture	D60XX
Single crown	Implant	Abutment fixed partial denture	D60XX

Categories group their code numbers into subcategories. Subcategories can be subdivided even further to make procedure determination easier. Maxillofacial prosthetics has no subcategory.

Category VIII has been shoehorned into the CDT code because this category of service was not recognized when the first code set was published in 1969. Emerging modalities of implant treatment show up in the subdivision to implant-supported prosthetics where there are a number of procedure codes from which to select a restoration (Table 2.7). In this instance, the CDT code differentiates between abutment-supported and implant-supported restorations.

CDT code categories are useful to visualize where a procedure best fits where there are number of possible choices. The appropriate code can be in different CDT categories. There are different CDT codes to report a single crown on a natural tooth and a crown on a natural tooth that supports a fixed partial denture. There are different CDT codes to report a single crown on a natural tooth and a crown on an implant-supported abutment (Table 2.8). These codes are not interchangeable. Application of the correct code hastens proper adjudication and payment of the claim.

The moribund subcategory, tests and examinations, promises to resurge with the introduction of diagnostic codes, treatment outcome, and alternative benefit payment systems to the dental care mix (Table 2.9). An emphasis on diagnosis moves dental care delivery from a procedure-driven fee-for-service payment system to an outcome-driven bundled payment system, like in accountable care organizations. Tracking diagnosis suddenly becomes important for health and the pocket book.

Table 2.9 Category I Diagnostic.

	Tests and examinations
D04xx	Collection and preparation of saliva sample for laboratory diagnostic testing
D04xx	Analysis of saliva sample
D04xx	Genetic test for susceptibility of oral diseases
D04xx	Caries susceptibility tests
D06xx	Caries risk assessment and documentation, with a finding of low risk
D06xx	Caries risk assessment and documentation, with a finding of moderate risk
D06xx	Caries risk assessment and documentation, with a finding of high risk

Tests and examinations for caries and periodontal disease risk establish the baseline for risk-based treatment choices and anticipatory care. Standardized tests will need to be adopted and adapted. Caries risk instruments like caries management by risk assessment (CAMBRA) and Previser are validated tools. Genetic testing for periodontal disease susceptibility is coming to the fore.

What this means to the clinician is a new way to look at dental treatment. Perhaps the future tilts from a surgical perspective (dentist forte is cutting) to a medical perspective (dentist forte is diagnosis) with a financial reward for healthier patients that requires less care.

Exclusion and limitation

The dental benefit booklet for a given plan sets out the exclusions—those instances where no benefit is available. One instance is the congenitally missing lateral incisor. While this can't be contested that a loss of the deciduous tooth requires restoration by an implant-supported crown or other procedures, the fact that the succedaneous tooth is congenitally missing often makes the replacement not a benefit. The exclusion is clearly stated in the benefit book. So, to entreat for obvious need runs up against a clear exclusion of a benefit, and the patient is left to pay for the procedure up to the allowed amount. This is a perfect illustration of where a predetermination of benefit is important for both the patient and the provider to get a clear understanding of the benefit.

Limitation

Dental benefit companies frequently put a limitation on a treatment code. That is, a benefit for a procedure is allowed under certain circumstances. For instance, scale and root plane is a definitive treatment that involves the instrumentation of the exposed root surface. This can be challenging for the clinician and painful to the patient. Some plans allow benefits for no more than two quadrants of scale and root plane on the same day. Another common example of a limitation is to benefit a crown lengthening procedure that requires a flap and bone removal when enough time has elapsed to heal before the crown impression.

The existence of a limitation of benefit supports the notion to predetermine benefits prior to treatment that's not an emergency or puts the patient in jeopardy of assuming a financial balance larger than expected.

Frequency limitation

This can mean the time interval between the same procedures. Following the scale and root plane example, there is usually a time interval between the initial and a second completed scale and root plan treatment.

One conundrum occurs with the frequency limitation for radiographs. Let's say that for a benefit there is a 60-month frequency limitation on a full series of films. That is, the benefit is paid only outside of this time period, and the patient is responsible for the cost of the treatment inside the time period. Let's also say that the dentist submits a claim for the treatment rendered knowing that it doesn't meet the frequency limitation and the patients pay the balance. The question is, does the benefit clock begin at the first series of films, or does it reset at the second set of films that are not a benefit?

Narrative for exclusion, limitation, and frequency

The example of an exclusion, limitation, and frequency limitation leads to the narrative. There are cases where the course of treatment takes the clinician outside of the CDT code descriptor or the dental plan benefit definition. A narrative can tip the balance. This is effective if the plan or policy is open to interpretation. It is not effective if the plan clearly excludes the benefit. So the narrative is a probable losing argument for the implant replacing a congenitally missing tooth but a probable winning argument for a repeat scale and root plane on a pregnant patient.

Dental plans often require a narrative to accompany a claim. The narrative supplements and supports the CDT code submitted. In addition, each category of the CDT code contains a Dx999—Unspecified, by report code—that requires a narrative to describe the procedure.

Be concise and succinct. Clearly describe the procedure and why the Dx999 or the other code is not adequately described in any other code. You should remember that a processor reads the narrative and a report written with condescension—patronizing superiority—is counterproductive to establish a relationship of understanding.

A short narrative can be inserted into Box 35 of the claim form. A longer narrative is submitted as an attachment.

Electronic claim submission

Practice management software systems that support electronic transactions are adept at populating the claim fields from the dental record. These systems generate a number of reports to track electronic claim submission. The validation report is to review before the send button is pushed. The transmission report confirms that the clearinghouse has received the report. The payer report confirms the claim's receipt by the third-party payer with information as to whether the claim is rejected, is denied, or requires more information.

Clearinghouse

A dental claim clearinghouse is the electronic link between dental management software and dental plans. The service is offered by a number of parties at a number of price points. The clearinghouse software provides a bridge to management software. In addition to dental claim transactions, a clearinghouse often offers other services like eligibility and benefits, claim status, electronic attachment, debit and credit card processing, and EOB report retrieval from dental plans.

Many dental benefit companies offer services to their providers for electronic claim transaction, electronic predetermination, claim tracking, EOB, ERA, and electronic funds transfer. The service supports only their claims and not the claims from other benefit companies. The service is as efficient as a clearinghouse plus it is free—there is no charge for the service.

Electronic attachment

To electronically attach a narrative, radiograph, treatment note, or periodontal chart to a claim streamlines document management and improves administrative processes. One company that provides this service is the NEA FastAttach® that matches claims to the attachment and eliminates the wait time normally associated with a request for additional documentation.

Code Maintenance Committee

There comes a time when a policy or document needs to be amended, revised, removed, or added. One example of a major addition is the implant code category. Clarity of intent is often achieved by small, nuance, continual change. To effect these enhancements is the essence of the Code Maintenance Committee (CMC).

The ADA's Council on Dental Benefit Programs (CDBP) is charged to maintain the CDT code. CDBP established the CMC to deliberate and vote on CDT code requests. The CMC convenes yearly. Accepted changes are incorporated into an updated version effected on January 1 of each year.

Any individual dentist, study club, specialty organization, manufacturer, technology company, or institution may request a CDT procedure code revision, addition, or deletion. Requests are submitted to the CMC on the official Action Request Form that is placed on the CMC timeline to be considered for discussion (Table 2.10). It can take up to 2 years for a request to be incorporated into the CDT code.

The CMC seeks to ensure that all the relevant stakeholders have an active role to evaluate and vote on the code set (Table 2.11). The CMC is comprised of five representatives from the ADA, one from each dental specialty, one from each

Table 2.10 Code Maintenance Committee timeline.

Event	Date
Closing date for request	November 1st
Code Maintenance Committee meets	February–March following year
CMC decision	April
ADA.org posted for public information	April
CDT manual prepared	May for following year
CDT code effective	January

Table 2.11 Code Maintenance Committee membership.

	Code Maintenance Committee (21 members)
1	American Dental Association (five members)
2	Academy of General Dentistry
3	American Dental Education Association
4	American Association of Endodontists
5	American Academy of Oral and Maxillofacial Pathology
6	American Academy of Oral and Maxillofacial Radiology
7	American Association of Oral and Maxillofacial Surgeons
8	American Association of Orthodontists
9	American Academy of Pediatric Dentistry
10	American Academy of Periodontology
11	American College of Prosthodontists
12	American Association of Public Health Dentistry
13	America's Health Insurance Plans
14	Blue Cross and Blue Shield Association
15	Centers for Medicare and Medicaid Services
16	Delta Dental Plans Association
17	National Association of Dental Plans

third-party payer organizations, and one each from the Academy of General Dentistry and the American Dental Education Association for a total of 21 voting members.

Every revision, addition, or deletion affects multiple stakeholders. A nuanced change of language or a wholesale change requires thoughtful consideration with the dental health outcome of the patient foremost. CDT codes do not address specific proprietary protocols that promise superior outcomes or specific tools to accomplish a procedure. A request is concise, reasoned, and supported by sound research conducted by reputable sources. With this in mind, the CDT code contains many changes, additions, and deletions each year, and successful requests have certain features in common (Table 2.12).

Table 2.12 CDT code request features.

Request	Hints for request
New code	Document clinical efficacy
New code	No reference to trade name
New code	Taught in dental institutions
New code	Literature to support change
New code	No reference to technique or protocol
New code	No reference to instrumentation
New code	Supported by specialty organizations
All requests	Concise and clear without ambiguity
All requests	Accurately document procedure
All requests	Not to unbundle or fragment procedure
All requests	Multiple requests for the same procedure

Nondentist provider

The CDT code set applies to providers and claim submission nationwide. It is based on the precept that the dentist is the provider of the service. The CDT code recognized nondentist providers when it added under Category I—"Diagnostic," the subcategory of "Pre-diagnostic Services." In this subcategory, two codes appear: screening of a patient and assessment of a patient. These two codes are specific to nondentist providers to bill for a limited screening and assessment.

However, the dental practice law in some states is evolving to recognize the nondentist provider and allows the nondentist provider to perform certain dental direct services without the supervision of a dentist. The CDT code will soon evolve to address these changes to dental care delivery.

One dental benefit claim wrinkle coming to the fore is the advent of unsupervised dental hygiene practice and the midlevel provider. Nondentist providers who submit a dental claim for their services directly to a third-party payer require a change in the participating provider contract (to include nondentist provider) basket of goods (procedures allowed by statute) and a realignment of the CDT code to recognize the nondentist provider (other than the prediagnostic screening).

For instance, in Colorado, the unsupervised dental hygienist is allowed to evaluate, diagnose, and create a treatment plan for a dental hygiene-related service like scaling and root planing. But the CDT code limits all evaluation codes to be performed by a dentist. The descriptor for the prediagnostic assessment and screening codes don't adequately describe and compensate for the evaluation service delivered. The Dx999 unspecified code may not attach a fee or a benefit to a service that would be a benefit if a dentist performed the same procedure. So what CDT code can be submitted by the unsupervised dental hygienist that accurately describes the service performed (bill for what you do), falls within an existing code, and allows the same benefit that a dentist receives for the same service?

In another instance, again in Colorado, a pending bill (HB 15-309) would allow the unsupervised dental hygienists to perform the interim therapeutic restoration (ITR) on both children and adults. However, the single CDT ITR code is for the primary dentition. How does the provider submit an ITR procedure for an adult patient?

The nondentist provider treating patients independent of a dentist presents an additional CDT code and benefit assignment challenge when put into the context of teledentistry, virtual dental home, and hub-and-spoke dental delivery models. In a fee-for-service system where multiple independent providers in this scenario deliver care to the same patient, what codes are used and who gets benefited? Is the capture and interpretation of a radiograph a separate code and charge? If so, who is benefited if the interpretation is done by multiple providers in the chain for the same incident of care?

There is certainly a lot of work ahead for the CMC to reconcile the changes occurring in dental care delivery throughout the 50 states.

Diagnosis code

A second set of codes for dentists to master is on the horizon. The CDT code reports a procedure—what is done. Diagnosis codes are to report a diagnosis—why it's done. This is increasingly important for dentists and dental practice as the health-care system moves toward measuring outcome rather than process. Is it more important to know whether the procedure is performed correctly or whether the right procedure is selected or whether the right procedure produced the desired outcome of reduced or managed disease?

There is no commonly accepted standardized terminology for oral diagnoses. The benefits of a common terminology to describe dental diagnosis are documentation of the type and frequency of conditions and outcome tracking. The value to track disease and treatment patterns is enormous. Risk-adjusted, cross-sectional, and temporal variations to access to health care, health-care quality, cost of care, and treatment effectiveness are what the dental profession aspires and the consumer expects. For the clinician in everyday practice, the diagnosis code hones diagnostic skills that emphasize the link between diagnosis and treatment. It moves the dentist from a treatment-centric view of the world to a diagnostic view with the horizon being better health outcome.

Given the need for information and knowledge management in dentistry to aggregate data for sophisticated quality improvement research, it can only be assumed that diagnostic terms in dentistry have come to stay. Anecdotal impressions entered into a paper record in a dental practice silo not connected to any other system will become archaic. Dental care will rely more heavily on evidenced-based care and population health outcomes based on the accumulated diagnostic data garnered from electronic dental record that's bridged to the patient's electronic health record.

ICD-10

Physicians and hospital already use diagnostic codes where it is embedded into the health record where HIPAA-covered entities that use electronic administrative transactions bill for services. The International Statistical Classification of Diseases and Related Health Problems 10th edition (ICD-10) covers more than 14,400 different codes and has been around for a century. The ICD-10 code sets breadth and granularity of ICD-10 that reflects advances in medicine and captures socioeconomic data, lifestyle-related problems, and the results of screening tests. These features create a robust database that will be valuable to the dental delivery system of the future.

Systematized Nomenclature of Dentistry (SNODENT) provides standardized terms for describing dental disease. It enables the capture, aggregation, and analysis of detailed oral health data.

Potential benefits include better communication among dentists, improved evidence-based practice, evaluation oral care outcomes, and the capability to measure adherence to standards of care.

SNODENT is an effort by the ADA to develop a controlled terminology to address the needs of clinical dentistry. The ADA, in collaboration with the College of American Pathologists, developed and incorporated SNODENT as a microglossary of SNOMED that's used in medicine. The ADA owns and maintains SNODENT and licenses its use.

EZCode diagnostic terminology has been integrated into the treatment plan module of the axiUm electronic health record. Several dental schools implemented the EZCode terminology where the next generation of clinician is being inculcated into terms of diagnosis. Future work will focus on refinement of the terms and strategies to enhance valid and efficient entry of terminology. EZCode has the promise of acceptance by all educational institutions with an open nonproprietary system. Elsbeth Kalenderian and her colleagues at Harvard School of Dental Medicine developed EZCode.

Boxes 29a, 29b, 34, and 34a in the ADA 2012 dental claim pave the way for diagnostic codes to populate the dental claim fields.

Conclusion

To understand the dental claim form and dental claim submission is not something to be delegated to a nonowner. The very lifeblood of your practice relies on the effective administrative system that's continually checked and monitored.

The participating provider agreement, ADA dental claim form, and the CDT code, which are the essential building blocks, were introduced that will keep you in good stead. The coming of diagnostic codes, the nondentist provider, and the payment systems other than fee-for-service will challenge the way of life for the independent solo private practitioner.

The learning in this chapter is not peripheral to the dental practice but funda-mental and essential. We're talking about dental practice not dental care. One must be both a master clinician and a master manager. One can't flourish without the other. There's no choice.

In a fee-for-service world where a provider is paid for every discrete service delivered, the importance to submit an accurate dental claim in an efficient system is the paramount feature to successful financial administration. This chapter introduced essential characteristics of a claim benefit system that assures smoother adjudication and faster payment of dental claims. Cash and cash flow are the lifeblood of the practice. Ignore this chapter at your peril.

CHAPTER 3

Dental benefits: Get it right

Michael M. Okuji

Delta Dental of Colorado, Denver, USA

Introduction

If you own a private practice, get dental claims right or suffer. If you're a partner in a group practice, get dental claims right or suffer. If you're the clinical director of a community health center, get dental claims right or suffer. Getting it right the first time on every transaction increases cash flow and minimizes administrative redundancy.

To get it right on the claim form means getting it right on the dental record, on the treatment plan, and into the financial ledger. This chapter points to the quirks of the CDT Code that throw you off and quagmires found on the claim form, claim submission, and claim appeal that mire the front office in endless frustration.

To get it right is not a trivial issue or an impediment to quality of care. To get it right is the lifeblood of a thriving business. To get it right on the claim form drives quality of care by insisting on the completeness of thought in the patient encounter and the precision required to record those thoughts in the patient record.

To delegate the design of the claims submission system is the surrender of control over the business. A dental business owner ignores this admonishment at their peril.

Get it right

The art of dentistry requires documentation of the diagnosis, treatment plan, and treatment that is so clear that anyone can read the dental record and know why, what, and how you performed the treatment. How much detail depends on how clear you intend to be.

The science of dentistry requires matching treatment rendered to the CDT Code. Because a dental procedure has nuances, not every procedure performed has an exact CDT Code match. Nevertheless, to be creative and add a personal procedure code or write a definition or engage in unbundling results in needless delay.

Dental Benefits and Practice Management: A Guide for Successful Practices, First Edition.
Edited by Michael M. Okuji.
© 2016 John Wiley & Sons, Inc. Published 2016 by John Wiley & Sons, Inc.

The business of dentistry requires a system that populates the dental claim and submits the claim with accuracy and efficiency. Accuracy counts because if all the elements of the dental claim are in place, the claim will fly through the auto-adjudication process. Most dental claims are auto-adjudicated by a computer and never seen by a reviewer. Claims that are clean are kicked out for review and action.

Participating provider agreement

To get it right means to understand the contractual agreement between the provider and the benefit company. The participating provider agreement is a binding business arrangement. The provider and the benefit company choose to enter into an agreement. Don't waste time trying to circumvent the clauses in the agreement you don't like. Just understand the rights and obligations that both parties make to one another to let business arrangement run smooth to accomplish the goals of each.

Fees

The fee arrangement is usually paramount for a provider. Fee-for-service is the norm for procedure reimbursement of the dental benefit world. Piecework is the standard by which most providers are paid—paid for each discrete procedure.

Fees are submitted and allowed. A submitted fee is the fee charged by the provider and is entirely at the provider's discretion. The manner in which the submitted fee for each procedure is derived is a hodgepodge method that usually boils down to the local average fee. The allowed fee is the maximum fee for each procedure that the provider agrees to accept. The allowed fee is usually lower than the submitted fee although claim data show that some provider's submitted fee is lower than the allowed fee. The dental benefit is calculated from the allowed fee. The allowed fee can be the filed fee or the fee schedule.

The allowed filed fee is the fee for each procedure that a provider submits and the benefit company accepts. The allowed filed fee is the one from which a benefit is determined. The mix of acceptable filed fees is subject to a proprietary algorithm.

The fee schedule is a list of allowed fees for each procedure. The fee schedule is set by the benefit company and is accepted or rejected by the provider. The provider accepts or rejects the fee schedule as a whole and can't pick and choose which fees they accept.

There are occasions when a benefit company negotiates filed fees or the fee schedule with a provider. This occurs when a benefit company wants to incentivize a provider to join because there is a lack of providers in the region or the benefit company wants to build a provider network for competitive reasons. Negotiated higher fees aren't evergreen and can revert to the base fee.

Utilization

More important than the fee is the utilization. That is how many patients are available and how many times they do actually access service. It does a provider no service to negotiate a high fee, even up to the list price, where there are no patients. One value-add to be in a provider network is the exposure to a large member base. The opportunity to negotiate a higher fee when there are no patients compounds the provider's view that other benefit companies have low fees when, in fact, the higher fee's promise of more revenue is illusionary.

Utilization review

The participating provider agreement allows for a utilization review process. It is not a function to be debated. The utilization review process varies from company to company. Utilization review of a provider network is often required by the insurance commissioner or other regulatory bodies to comply with state statutes.

Utilization review is a retrospective process. It looks back in time for patterns of practice that are significantly different from their provider's peers. There are a number of trends that are reviewed and the mix changes over time (Table 3.1). A provider that seems to be following aberrant practice patterns may be placed on focused review for closer monitoring and be required to submit documentation, not required from other providers, for certain procedures.

Audits sometimes follow a utilization review that falls outside of standard deviation(s) from peers. An audit can be an in-depth, ongoing review of dental claim trends or a desk audit where the actual financial ledger, appointment book, and dental record are reviewed. In either case, being different is not to be bad. It just means to be different.

Prospective utilization review

A more dynamic process is the prospective utilization review that utilizes enormous dental claim datasets plus other datasets to project future treatment behavior. Rather than look back at past trends, prospective utilization review looks forward to project future provider utilization trend. This is akin to a credit score that prospectively projects the credit holder's payment behavior.

Table 3.1 Utilization review examples.

Utilization pattern	Reason
Every extraction is surgical	Not substantiated in the dental record
Seven vertical bitewings on every visit	No frequency limitation
Crown replacement	At 5-year frequency limitation
Restoration on a missing tooth	Clerical error or fraud
Repeated treatment	Multiple patients billed under one
Root plane and scale	In the absence of periodontal disease

Table 3.2 Machine learning objectives.

Technique applied to	Predictive problem solved
Fuzzy logic	Health care
Neural network	Biomedical
Cognitive process	Big data
Decision support	Business
Decision tree	Education
Expert system	Cyber security
Evolutionary algorithm	Software process
Markov model	Cost estimation
Probabilistic reasoning	Risk management
Ranking algorithm	
Reasoning model	
Recommender system	
Swarm intelligence	

Large claim datasets and access to other datasets enable robust and sophisticated computer algorithms to become a predictive learning tool with machine learning capability using techniques like fuzzy logic and neural networks that continually learn through pattern recognition, without being explicitly programed, emerging patterns of clinical behavior (Table 3.2).

Fuzzy logic is used to variably control a traffic signal to optimize traffic flow rather than set intervals of time. Even rice cookers use fuzzy logic to monitor moisture, heat, and time to make fluffy rice. Epidemiologists use machine learning to predict disease patterns and prevalence in populations.

Utilization review for most providers is invisible and a nonissue. For those providers who come into focused utilization review, the dental record stands as the bulwark against a claim of abusive practice. Far beyond its use to detect fraud, waste, and abuse, prospective utilization review holds the promise to improve quality of care and the patient experience.

Quality assurance audit

The audit is different from utilization review. The authority for a third-party payer to conduct a dental office audit can arise from a state law like the California Knox-Keene Act that regulates managed health-care plans in the state or the state insurance commissioner. Another authority to audit a dental office is through the contractual language of the participating provider agreement.

Quality assurance audits are based on the notion of consumer protection. The purpose enables the dental plan to demonstrate to state regulators that its network of providers provides quality care to its members and is fiscally responsible and sound. The dental office audit can be a physical assessment of equipment, radiographic safety, emergency service provisions, and Occupational Safety and Health Administration (OSHA) compliance.

Quality assurance audits can be for dental records review through an office audit of the dental records. State law and federal HIPAA privacy rule recognize the right of third-party payers to access the health records of its members, and this information can be legitimately reviewed for payment for treatment and assuring quality of care. Certain patterns of practice raise questions on the standard of care. For instance, is it the standard of care to take a radiographic series on every child on every visit even in the absence of caries risk history? What if a radiograph is nondiagnostic or lacks an image at all? What if the clinician believes they are at risk to miss disease unless a radiograph is taken at every opportunity?

In the case of the recovery of payments made to dentists, the participating provider agreement or the dentist handbook explains the terms in which a requested reimbursement may be recovered including a set-off amount that is deducted from subsequent payments to the dentists.

Appeal and dispute resolution

There are avenues to disagree with the outcome of claim adjudication, utilization review, or an audit. The participating provider agreement states the mechanism and time frame for the appeal and the dispute resolution process. State law is followed for benefit appeals.

Self-funded plans are governed by federal law and are exempt from state insurance laws. This can mean a difference in how the coordination of benefit is adjudicated and the application of any state prompt payment law. Employee Retirement Income Security Act (ERISA) plans are self-funded plans where the employer assumes the financial risk of the plan. Self-funded plans are most often administered by a dental benefit company that acts as the administrator of the dental benefit but carry no financial risk. To get it right is to remember that a dental benefit company that takes financial risk can change a claim in favor of the member or a benefit category (add a second fluoride application) without consulting the employer (the money comes from the benefit company). But a dental benefit company can't change a claim in favor of a member (like pay and educate for an EPO plan) or add a service (add a second fluoride) because the administration of the program and the financial risk rest with the employer (it's their money).

Appeal preparation

The best preparation to bring a case for appeal includes reference to the provider handbook, *Evidence of Coverage* (EOC), the dental claim, the evidence of benefit (EOB), and the documentation from the patient's dental record. These resources provide the basis for the appeal or dispute including the language for applying an exclusion or limitation. Highlight the specific passages you reference that support your case and display the misinterpreted basis of the denial. To get it right is to know that a disputed claim from a dental company operating in multiple states may process claims state by state. Don't dispute a California claim for treatment in Colorado even if the companies share a name.

Audits, appeals, and disputes are sometimes the result of clerical error or acts of goodwill or bad practice habits. While most dentists rely on managers in their office to oversee the administration of the practice, the ultimate responsibility for error resides with the owner of the practice even if others made the error. I'm reminded of Captain Robert J. Kelly who commanded the USS Enterprise when it ran aground in San Francisco Bay—Captain Kelly took responsibility even though the ship was in the control of the port pilot when it hit the sandbar. Financial recovery of losses due to misconduct under the guise of clerical error is not recoverable through property insurance coverage if it is deemed insurance fraud.

Termination

The participating provider agreement allows bilateral termination for cause or without cause. In either case, get it right and manage the termination of the agreement.

Termination isn't done in secrecy. Some state statutes require the benefit company to send notification of provider termination from the network to all members affected to alert them of the change of status.

Manage misinformation. To the members, the patients, what they hear is that they have no dental benefit if they continue to see the terminated provider. In the case of an exclusive provider dental plan (EPO), it is true that benefits will no longer be available for care at a non-par provider. But in other plan designs, benefits will continue after plan termination but the amount of benefit will be less and the patient portion more.

To get it right on a termination, determine what plan designs the patient carries. If it's one that allows payment (at a reduced rate) to a non-par provider, then the choice is to embark on a public relations campaign to alert the patients of the new par status but the same great care, or adjust the patient portion of the procedure fee as to be a nonissue for the patient (i.e., they have the same out-of-pocket expense before and after termination). Manage expectations and you get it right.

Summary

Hints to get it right are easy to do when taken separately but difficult when taken as a series of procedures. To get it right on a consistent and ongoing basis seems so daunting as to give up entirely on the endeavor. I would counter that it's the business we've chosen. We should be the best at what we do (Table 3.3).

Internalize the CDT Code for just the 30 most common procedures delivered. It's the common language for dental claims.

Be a master clinician that includes being the master of the patient record. It's not just to notate information for a dental claim. The clinical record, the chart note and treatment plan, is the only written record of what was done and why. The chart note should be as all-inclusive or brief as needed to clearly tell the story of the visit to another dentist that only has the chart note from which to refer.

The billing ledger is separate from the clinical record, and the information that populates it must match both the clinical record and the appointment book.

Table 3.3 Summarize handy hints.

	Handy hints
1 CDT Code book	Select 25 top codes and internalize each word
2 Clinical record	Memorialize what you do for the next dentist
3 Billing ledger	Matches clinical record and appointment book
4 Claim	Actual procedure(s) submitted
5 Cross-check	Multiple persons submit claims and payments
6 System	Implement an administrative system that cross-checks
7 Manage	The owner is the quality assurance

The clinical record must be made available to the patient. Don't put the ledger with the clinical record.

The dental claim includes the procedure actually performed and not the procedure that's expected to be paid. The dental claim includes those procedures that are not expected to be paid as a dental benefit. Submit for what you do.

The cross-check has multiple personnel administering the claim and payment process to assure cross-functionality and quality assurance. If the front office has a single person, then the owner becomes the cross-check. Less treatment and more administration for the solo dentist but that's what business owners have to do.

The system is developed and implemented by the dentist, not the office administrator. The dentist is the manager that sets the policy and procedures and is ultimately responsible for quality assurance. Policy and procedures are written documents that make up the desktop procedure book.

Dentist and dental plan design

To make sense of dental benefit design, it is useful to think of dentist and plan. A dentist has a designation and the plan has a designation. Together, they determine the amount of benefit available to the patient.

A dentist that chooses to enter into participating provider agreement is called participating or par. A dentist that chooses not to enter into an agreement is called nonparticipating or non-par. A par dentist is listed in the directory and the patient benefit is computed from the allowed fee amount. The positive aspect for a par is access to a large patient pool and the positive aspect for the member is a ceiling on fees. A non-par dentist is not listed in a directory.

A dental plan pays different benefits to a par and non-par dentist. An open-panel plan is where a patient can select a par or a non-par dentist for services and be reimbursed at some level. Most often, a par dentist has a higher benefit than a non-par dentist. In a closed-panel plan, a member that selects a par provider for services has a dental benefit. In a closed-panel plan, a member that selects a non-par for services has no benefit and not reimbursed for any service. Another name for a closed-panel plan is exclusive panel organization (EPO). Affordable Care Act on-exchange dental plans are closed panel that reimburse only par dentists.

Dental plan contract

The dental plan member, usually through their employer, has a separate contract between the benefit company and the employer. The EOC that is provided to the employees sets out the terms of the specific benefit plan and summarizes the benefits, exclusions, and limitations.

The EOC sets out the terms of the dental benefit to the member and not to limit the treatment decisions between the patient and their dentist. Only the patient and their dentist decide the course of treatment. The dental benefit is to assist in the payment of certain dental services and not to cover all services or even all needed services.

Of course, some patients elect only a treatment that is a covered benefit even if their dentist recommends a different course of treatment, for instance, giving a recommendation for prophylaxis every 3 months instead of every 6 months for a patient at higher periodontal risk like a pregnant patient. This is a situation where trust and good communication between the patient and dentist come into play. Getting it right means to understand the limitations and exclusions in the EOC and anticipate answers and provide solutions.

Dental claim process

Benefit eligibility

To get it right is to put benefit eligibility first in the administrative process queue. Is the patient currently eligible for benefits or is there a waiting period to extinguish? A new waiting period for an existing patient may occur if the patient's dental plan changes. So an eligible patient who changes plans next month may incur a new waiting period even if the same benefit company issues the new plan.

While many patients keep the same job and maintain their same dental benefits for years, other patients drift in and out of coverage. For instance, hourly workers who must maintain a minimum number of working hours per month to keep their dental benefits may have an episodic coverage over a calendar year— the same as patients covered under a COBRA plan who have month-to-month eligibility.

Use online tools to verify eligibility on the morning of treatment. This is the fastest and most accurate way to verify eligibility. Eligibility can be verified online before or after the benefit company's working hours. Eligibility verification is a standard operating procedure written into the desktop procedure. Eligibility verification by telephone wastes administrative time and resources. Avoid the telephone at all cost. The call is apt to be on hold longer than an online search,

Table 3.4 Eligibility information.

Source	Eligibility information
Dental plan ID card	Companies have multiple plans and designs
Enrollee ID number	Plans assigned unique number not Social Security Number
Dental plan handbook	Primary information source
Date of birth	Important in dual insurance
Other dental insurance	Coordination of benefits
	Enter even if patient does not intend to submit a claim
Primary custody of child	Financial planning
Student status	Plans coverage for students up to age 26

the call is not a guarantee of eligibility status, and there's always the off chance of a miscommunication—I heard, she said, scenario.

Eligibility records are uploaded from the employer files to the benefit company files frequently—even daily. Print out the eligibility verification for the record. This step is especially critical for cases with a high cost attached or for patients at risk for falling out of eligibility. The administrative practice to call in the morning and print out the status saves countless hours and dollars. This step eliminates one source of front-end administrative error that causes great patient dissatisfaction and loss of more time and money on the back end.

The sources for eligibility information start with the dental plan ID card, enrollee ID number, and date of birth of the insured and patient—in the case of a dependent, coordination of benefit information and student status (Table 3.4).

Evidence of coverage

A state-mandated document is the EOC that describes the benefits covered, exclusions, limitations, deductibles, and co-payment or coinsurance. The EOC supplements the online information and is more detailed. Important information is the scope of benefits, limitations (e.g., 60-month crown replacement), and exclusions (e.g., restoration of congenitally missing teeth). If there is a limitation, a predetermination, with a thoughtful narrative that focuses on the limitation, may be warranted. If a procedure is excluded, there is no benefit even in the case of dental need. Don't start an implant, abutment, and crown for an extracted retained deciduous maxillary lateral incisor without reading the EOC or, better yet, predetermine the case. It's not an emergency. The benefit is not a matter of the need to restore the area. It's the contractual exclusion of the situation.

Coordination of benefit

It is common for two adults in a family to both have a dental plan that covers their dependent child. In this case, coordination of benefits comes into play with rules to determine which plan is the primary plan for the payment of benefit determination.

Table 3.5 Coordination of benefit rules.

	Rule		Coordination of benefit for dependent
1	Birthday rule		The parent whose birthday falls first in the calendar year is the primary plan for the dependent. If both parents have the same birthday, the plan in effect the longest is the primary plan
2	Custody rule	Primary	Plan of the parent with custody
3	Custody rule	Second	Plan of the spouse of the custodial parent
4	Custody rule	Third	Plan of the parent without custody
5	Custody rule	Fourth	Plan of the spouse of the parent without custody
6	Court ordered		Court order that specifies one parent is responsible for the dependent child's dental expenses
7	Working retiree		Active plan is primary and retiree plan secondary

The rules that govern coordination of benefits are the birthday rule, the custody rule, the court-ordered rule, and the working retiree rule (Table 3.5).

Coordination of benefit between a commercial dental benefit carrier and Medicaid poses a particularly sticky problem. Workers in low-wage industries are eligible for Medicaid benefits and may have commercial insurance too. They may have a monthly work schedule that fluctuates and pushes them in and out of insurance eligibility. The problem occurs because they prefer to use Medicaid dental benefits in lieu of the commercial plan. Commercial dental benefits carry a deductible and a co-payment for which the patient is responsible to pay. Medicaid dental benefits have neither a deductible nor a co-payment, and the member has no out-of-pocket cost. Of course, a member prefers to use their Medicaid dental benefit instead of their commercial benefit. But Medicaid is always the payer of last resort and pays only when there is no other source. So when a patient presents their Medicaid card for dental services instead of their commercial card, the state is on the hook for payment and the dentist is out of the balance. In the end, a time-consuming financial reckoning occurs.

Nonduplication of benefit

In the case of dual coverage and coordination of benefit, some companies invoke a nonduplication of benefit provision when a group elects this proviso. This means the secondary carrier pays the difference between what the primary carrier actually paid and what the secondary carrier would have paid if it were the primary carrier. So if the primary carrier pays 80% for a procedure and the secondary carrier normally covers 80% for the same procedure, the secondary carrier is not obligated to pay any benefit at all. Now, you might think the procedure should be covered 100% with no patient out-of-pocket cost and told the patient so. After all, the secondary carrier has to benefit 20% not 80% and is better off. But no, the nonduplication of service clause prohibits this calculation and there is 20% yet to be paid by the, now, irate patient.

Unbundled procedure

To unbundle a procedure is to break the procedure into distinct components and bill each component separately. For instance, an unbundled procedure is pulpal debridement and endodontic therapy. Unbundled procedure is crown preparation, laboratory fee, and crown restoration. In both cases, the pieces are part of the whole and billed as one procedure even if there is a separate CDT Code or a Dx999 is submitted.

Balance billing

The practice of balance billing is to charge a patient with dental benefits up to the provider's submitted charge rather than the allowed charge under the participating provider agreement. For instance, if the submitted amount is $125, the allowed amount is $100, and the procedure has an 80% benefit, the plan's benefit is $80 and the patient portion is $20. Any patient portion above $20 is balance billing (Table 3.6).

What occurs in the case of an extraordinary laboratory charge, or difficulty to achieve profound anesthesia, or the convenience to the patient for a same-day procedure that warrants a charge above the allowed fee? In most cases, the CDT Code includes certain features of a procedure like anesthesia, temporization, laboratory fee, and an anatomic and natural restoration. The CDT Code doesn't include different subcategories of D27xx porcelain, ceramic substrate, to account for different materials or fabrication technique, so to charge different fees for different materials under the same code is not allowed. The CDT Code doesn't recognize the tool or technique used to achieve the result whether it is a laser or CAD–CAM technology. A convenience fee for the use of a particular tool is not a recognized CDT Code procedure and not chargeable to the patient. To unbundle a procedure and charge for the extra step is not allowable.

To get it right is to bill for what is done. That can be a D92xx inhalation of nitrous oxide or non-intravenous moderate sedation for the anxious patient or a Dx999 unspecified procedure, by report, for an unusual service outside of the normal steps for the procedure. To charge a patient and not bill to the benefit carrier is deceptive and not allowed by contract. In those cases where an unusual step has been taken, get it right, submit the procedure as a Dx999, and attach a persuasive narrative. That's the key.

Table 3.6 Balance billing.

Balance bill	Dollar	Reason
Patient portion—not allowed	45	Balance billed amount
Patient portion	20	Allowed balance
Dental benefit	80	80% of allowed fee
Allowed fee	100	Maximum allowed fee
Submitted fee	125	Dentist fee

Noncovered service

The term noncovered service applies to a procedure that is not a plan benefit, and the maximum payment for the procedure is limited to the allowed fee. By contract, noncovered services are denied and the member pays up to the allowed fee. In states with statutes that prohibit the maximum allowable fee on noncovered services, the dentist may charge any fee without restriction.

Upcode

To upcode is to submit for a more expensive procedure than the procedure actually performed. The single extraction codes (D7xxx) are prone to upcode scrutiny. It's expected that a mix of extraction codes will be submitted. It is suspicious when only surgical extractions (D72xx) are submitted without any simple extraction (D71xx).

The same can be said of the surgical removal of root tips, extraction, and extraction of coronal remnants. The surgical removal requires removal of soft tissue and bone, while a D71xx extraction doesn't require those steps. Does the clinical record support a surgical removal of root tips or more closely describe an extraction? Does the clinical record support extraction or the removal of deciduous teeth coronal remnants? To get it right, the clinical record, including radiographs, substantiates the procedure.

Deny and disallow

Dental plans use the terms deny and disallow with specific meanings. Some submitted procedures are not paid and the terms deny and disallow are applied. Deny means the procedure is not payable by the dental plan but chargeable to the patient with the maximum charge, in some cases, limited to the allowed amount. Disallow means the procedure is not payable by the dental plan and not chargeable to the patient. The specific reason for a deny or disallow decision is coded on the explanation of benefits (EOB) report.

To get it right is to remember that just because a procedure is listed in the CDT Code doesn't mean the procedure is a covered benefit and automatically eligible for a benefit.

Appeal a claim determination

When a claim is denied, is disallowed, or is just not properly adjudicated by the terms of the EOC, an appeal is appropriate. Each company sets out their specific appeal rights for the dentists. The appeal is required to be a written appeal with supporting documentation that did not accompany the original claim, like a narrative or supplemental radiographs. The appeal must be submitted within a certain time period and the adjudication of the appeal returned within a certain time period, usually 45 days. It is incumbent upon the dentist to walk the reviewing consultant through the steps in order for the consultant to see their side of the story to approve the benefit for the patient.

One reason to uphold a denied claim upon appeal is a dental record that does not support the facts of the appeal. This is usually based on the lack of adequate notation in the dental record. An extraction is notated in the dental record as a surgical extraction without further elaboration. The dental record entry seems to be for benefit coding rather than the health record. The assertion that certain steps are always taken in a surgical extraction and need not be notated is not defensible for a claim appeal nor is it the standard of care.

Electronic services

To get it right and get it fast go hand in hand when it comes to dental claim submission and benefit payment. There is absolutely no reason for a dentist not to use all of the electronic administrative tools available for eligibility, predetermination, claim submission, attachments, and payment. Electronic tools drastically cut the adjudication time in those cases where additional information is requested, an appeal submitted, or a dispute is settled.

Telephone calls are a waste of time and nonbinding. There are too many ways for a simple telephone conversation to be misconstrued. To build a patient estimate and financial plan based on telephone call is folly. While the dental office can blame the patient's benefit carrier for the misinformation leading to an underestimate, it's the patient that bears the unexpected bill and the dentist that bears the brunt of a dissatisfied customer.

Eligibility

Eligibility through a website is common for most benefit carriers. If the dental benefit is an important consideration for the patient to seek treatment, their eligibility status should be established prior to their first visit. Many plans have waiting periods before eligibility is established (like CHP+ medically necessary orthodontics) or waiting periods before certain services are eligible (12-month wait for a crown). This isn't to say that a patient shouldn't embark on recommended immediately necessary treatment prior to dental benefit eligibility, but rather they should know beforehand the risks and make a reasoned decision for themselves.

Predetermination

Electronic predetermination takes only days to process even when attachments are requested. For some claims, auto-adjudication takes seconds, mere seconds. To say that a predetermination takes up to 30 days comes from an office that submits a paper claim.

Predetermination usually means the estimate of the allowed fee and benefit payment if the patient remains eligible and the maximum has not been reached. A disconnect occurs when a predetermined claim for a crown is denied payment because the endodontist submitted the root canal claim first that extinguished the maximum dollars available for the year.

Some administrative consultants view the predetermination of treatment as lowering case acceptance because the patient is the most motivated to begin treatment immediately after the diagnosis is made and engaged with their dentist. This is an administrative choice by a business consultant, not a treatment choice by a dentist.

With the numerous permutations of dental plans, a prudent dentist will predetermine intended procedures for certain categories of service. While prophylaxis and examination coverage ascertained by telephone may be tolerable, a crown in the $1500 range may warrant a predetermination. This dispels any doubt on limitation, frequency, exclusion, and benefit. The time interval between the diagnosis and the treatment date for a crown is usually enough time to electronically predetermine the benefit and get it right the first time.

Claim submission

Once a claim is predetermined, it takes very little administrative time to input the date of service than electronically submit the claim for payment.

There is a secret incantation to magically get a claim paid. But there are a number of everyday steps (written into the desktop process) that assists faster adjudication, proper reimbursement of services, and prompt payment. Incomplete or erroneous patient and provider information is the number one culprit for a delay in the processing of a claim (Table 3.7). Are all the identifiers for the patient and provider correct?

Electronic funds transfer

A predetermined electronic claim need only have the treatment date entered and the send button pushed to electronically to begin the adjudication process that takes place usually that same day. Some clearinghouse process claims in real time and others process in a batch at the end of the day. The benefit company sends the reimbursement to the bank via electronic funds transfer (EFT) and your account credited.

Table 3.7 Common field errors.

Who	What	How	Why
Patient	Birthdate	xx/xx/201x	If dependent is the patient
Patient	ID	Employer designated ID	Not Social Security Number
Provider	Employee	Billing vs. treating dentist	Group practice
Provider	Tooth	Crown placed on extraction site	#3 vs. #14
Provider	Date service	Preparation vs. seat	December 20th vs. January 10th
Provider	CDT Code	Obsolete code	D1203 topical fluoride
Benefit company	Address	One company can have multiple billing addresses	Administrative not processing address
Benefit company	Subsidiary	One company can have multiple subdivisions	California for a Colorado company plan

Only dental offices demand a paper check. There is no sense to have others hold your money when you can have it in your bank account today. The principal source of delay and irritation for claim processing and payment is the use of paper. Paper processing of the claim involves the queue to mail from the office, mail delivery, queue to open and scan, batch queue to mail, and mail delivery. The paper process is time consuming and is exacerbated if there is a request for more information—all through the same laborious paper trail. The move away from paper to electronic transactions saves a considerable amount of time and wrests cost savings from the administrative expense of running a practice.

Quick payment receipt is a sign of a healthy financial system. The explanation of benefit or electronic remittance advice allows the office to get it right when it comes time to reconcile the patient's financial ledger. It's here that errors are caught and rectified. In fact, if all the other electronic steps are followed, the EFT should be the last payment step and the patient's ledger is zeroed out.

Claim filing tips

These issues occur frequently with tips on how to manage them. Internalize the tips and write the desktop procedure. This effort goes a long way to get it right every time, every day.

1 Most delays occur because of missing or inaccurate information. Fill in all the dental claim fields. Be consistent with the words. The patient may always go by the name Anne but is listed on the benefit record as Annette.

2 Check eligibility on the morning of the appointment. Doing so electronically allows the process to begin prior to the benefit company opens for office hours. The dental plan has a new waiting period to be extinguished because the benefit company is the same but the employer changed benefit plans. The patient is ineligible because they didn't work enough hours last month. The new dental plan is an EPO, limited network plan, that won't pay for any service outside of the network and the office doesn't participate. All of these are easily avoidable by insuring accurate claim form information and confirming eligibility on the day of service.

3 Know the dental claim requirements of the three largest benefit payers to your office by the number of claims. Have their provider handbook readily accessible. Do they require an attachment for certain procedures on the first submission of the claim? Or do they routinely detach and discard attachments (yes they do this) and send a request for additional information as needed? Don't waste time and resources by attaching radiographs if they won't be scanned and filed on the first round. Their policy is that it saves the dental office time from wasting company's resources to scan and file documents that aren't needed for adjudication.

4 Legible, accurate, and complete dental claims fly through auto-adjudication by a computer and reviewer processing. Avoid handwritten paper claims. Don't be surprised that in the near future, paper claims are put at the back of a queue and paper checks are batched for mailing once per month and a service charge is assessed. Banks do it—so will benefit companies. Don't try to set up a personal protocol because it's easier for the dental office (i.e., attaching radiographs to every crown case). Go with the flow. Don't try to be different.

5 Use electronic services as much as possible. It's fast, effective, and efficient. It saves people time and lowers administrative overhead. Repeated calls to a customer service line to obtain the entire book of benefits are a bad business practice. There are other more efficient ways to obtain this information.

6 Frustration with the dental claim process often times starts with the dental office. Populate the dental claim with good data. It's good for the patient and the practice. Refresh patient data frequently. Personal information changes: address, marital status. Employment information changes: employer, hourly worker. Dental plans change even if from the same employer and the same dental company. Open enrollment gives choice and there may be a new waiting period, deductible amount, or exclusive network plan.

7 Use the latest version of the ADA Dental Claim Form (J430D 2012). Include the current telephone number. Include a corporate contact number if another entity files your claims. Remember Box 35 remarks for unusual services. The billing dentist and treating dentist is accurate.

8 Only send radiographs if they are needed. Different companies have different policies. Know the policy of the top three payers in your office. Some companies automatically detach radiographs from the claim and discard the radiograph. It's simply too time consuming for them to scan and file unrequested radiographs. Never send a radiograph unless requested for the case. If a radiograph is requested, do send it via electronic attachment. Electronic attachments are received by the benefit carrier almost instantaneously and won't materially delay adjudication of a predetermination or a claim for payment. To mail a copy of a radiograph is wasteful and time consuming. To mail the original radiograph is foolish. Of course, radiographs must be of diagnostic quality with sharpness and contrast.

Oddly, radiographs are sometimes submitted that are distorted to the point that a tooth can't be discerned or, worse of all, an exposed radiograph with no tooth image at all. Digital panoramic, bitewing, and periapical views should be enlarged so that the viewer can readily interpret the radiograph. If a physical copy is mailed, orient the radiograph correctly with the dimple facing out if it's on a film or a right and left inscription if it's on paper. Radiographs that are faxed come out too dark to read (who faxes anymore?). The convention is the viewer is looking from the outside of the arch.

Use quality photo paper for the best image. Mount the radiographs securely with the patient name, practice name and address affixed, and the date imaged.

Don't send a film in a coin envelope and expect someone else to orient the radiographs correctly and keep track.

Panoramic films are optimal for oral surgery and as an orientation to a complex case. The panoramic film isn't diagnostic for restorative, endodontic, and periodontal surgery cases.

The obvious errors that delay claim adjudication are assigning the wrong radiograph to a patient or attaching a radiograph that fails to show the treatment area. Preoperative radiographs are essential to document diagnosis and to justify treatment. A working length endodontic radiograph or a crown's final seat radiograph doesn't really justify the treatment.

Finally, don't expect radiographs to be returned even if a stamp-addressed envelope is enclosed for that purpose.

9 The periodontal chart is an essential entry into the dental record. The periodontal chart is considered a part of the comprehensive oral evaluation for the new and established patient and the periodic oral evaluation for the established patient. Of course, the periodontal chart is central to the comprehensive periodontal evaluation for the new or established patient.

Failure to adequately document a periodontal chart for these evaluations is considered below the standard of care. A paper-based chart is copied and mailed or scanned and attached to an electronic claim. Entries to a paper periodontal chart tend to be cluttered or illegible.

A streamlined practice employs digital periodontal charting. A digital chart is clear and easily attached to an electronically claim. Features of a periodontal chart include six-point tooth readings, mobility, furcation, gingival attachment (or loss), and missing teeth.

It's recommended that a pocket greater than 3 mm is indicated by circling the tooth and not the pocket number. Highlighter pen or red ink interferes with scanned and faxed image.

A narrative goes a long way to substantiate the need for the periodontal procedure. Walk the reader through the diagnosis. In some cases, a narrative can be more persuasive than the periodontal chart and radiograph.

10 Narratives are powerful tools. They are often employed to explain procedures with covered benefits that are denied or disallowed, and the clinician feels it is improperly adjudicated.

Narratives are not for procedures that are expressly excluded in the patient's EOC booklet. Benefit exclusion in the EOC for replacement of congenitally missing teeth is never a benefit regardless of the need for restoration.

A narrative is the way for the clinician to describe the clinical situation that is not clear on a radiograph or is inadequately described in the CDT Code descriptor. It walks the reviewer through the diagnostic process. A short narrative description can be entered into Box 35 remarks. Longer narratives are sent via electronic attachment. Letter length narratives are best left to the appeal step of claim adjudication.

All narratives include the date of the narrative, date of the service or pre-determination, patient name, dentist name, and contact information. Type a narrative as handwritten narratives are all-too-often illegible. The narrative is clear, concise, and to the point. Radiographs, photographs, and charting clearly support and are congruent to the narrative.

Narratives are especially effective for fixed and removable restorative cases with complications and special needs. The narrative is specific to the case and is substantiated by the clinical record. It is not a general statement. To say a restoration is needed to restore the tooth to proper form and function isn't helpful. Boilerplate (standardized text) narratives are counterproductive, and the clinician looses credibility with each boilerplate submission.

The clinician always writes the narrative and never delegates writing to a nondentist. If a narrative is important to the case, it's important that a clinician writes it. A collegial tone is set to convey understanding and not intellectual superiority. A diatribe is never appropriate. Nor are unsubstantiated statements of superior quality of service or procedure.

Box 35 remarks and narratives are powerful tools to explain the clinical case for treatment not obvious in other records. Narratives make all the difference in the world on a close-call case. The more one writes narratives, the better one becomes at writing effective narratives. Don't give up.

11 Fillings and crowns fracture, and bridges sometimes fail prematurely and need replacement. For dental benefit adjudication, restorative procedures carry a replacement time frame. For amalgams and resins, it can be 24 months. For crowns and dentures, it can by 60 months. To submit a claim for a replacement within the time limitation for a restoration, it's good practice to document the clinical reason.

If the dental claim is for a patient of record, always enter the date of prior placement in Box 43 replacement of a prosthesis and reason for replacement in Box 35 remarks. Write a narrative attachment if a longer description is needed. If the dental claim is for a new patient, enter the date the patient entered the practice and the date of prior placement to the patient's best recollection. Use at least the year of prior placement, 2015, and not just say more than 5 years.

Some dental plans allow replacement of restorations in less than the minimum frequency if a different dentist or dental office does the replacement restoration. It's always recommended that a predetermination be obtained prior to replacing a restoration if it is not an emergency situation or the fee would cause issue if the benefit were not paid.

12 Dentistry doesn't have a standard of care based on a body of knowledge that is universally adopted by clinicians for the need for crown. Neither does dentistry employ diagnostic codes.

In the absence of diagnostic codes, documentation for the need for full or partial coverage crown is recommended. A decayed or otherwise damaged tooth can be restored by any number of different procedures. A careful clinician will document the diagnosis in the dental record and transfer that information to the dental claim.

Caries, undermined cusp, and fractured or missing cusp are documented through radiographs, photographs, or clinical notes. The diagnosis, treatment, and prognosis are recorded. Some claims to restore a damaged tooth with a crown are clear on their own merits. Others need more explanation. For instance, why a full-coverage crown on a molar and not a three-surface amalgam? Is it because a cusp is likely to fracture in the future and preemptive cusp coverage is the standard of care? Be prepared to defend the interpretation of the profession's standard of care.

Full coverage of all endodontic treated teeth is not an automatic basis for a benefit. Be prepared to support a full crown on a tooth with no existing restoration, small access opening, and sufficient tooth structure.

13 Technology advancement brings up the new phenomenon of the "convenience fee." If new technology allows the fabrication of a crown on the same day of the preparation, should a patient be charged for this convenience over other techniques? How is convenience submitted on a dental claim? One might say that it is clearly a benefit to the patient to save time and an additional fee is warranted for the convenience and to cover the cost of expensive technology. Others might say that the manner in which a crown is fabricated is part of the base fee.

A related technology-driven phenomenon is customization of ceramic crowns. Some types of ceramic crowns are fabricated from a single block of material and are typically used for posterior teeth where the monochromatic nature is not too much of an issue. Is the customization of this fabrication technique part of the procedure or an additional charge?

When it comes to the dental benefit, the notion of "submit for what you do" is appropriate. Submit the fee and adjudication follows. Remember we are talking about a participating provider that treats a covered member under a binding contractual agreement that is voluntarily entered.

14 The restorative foundation and crown buildup procedures (D29xx) draw a lot of attention. For some benefit plans, these procedures are considered part of the restoration. The core buildup comes under the most scrutiny because it is applied in cases to block out an undercut or to level the pulpal floor. The Box 35 remark or a narrative with diagrams can clearly explain the need for additional resistance or retention form without which the crown would just fall off. Again, the use of boilerplate (standardized text) is discouraged and using a description specific to the tooth is recommended.

15 Use the proper code for the procedure. Don't interchange two seemingly similar codes like the core buildup and the post and core. The post and core, either indirectly fabricated or prefabricated, requires an existing sealed root canal that can be shown in the preoperative film.

16 The definition of a fracture is fluid in the profession and, in some cases, inappropriately overused and inflated. A cusp that shears off exposing the

underlying dentin is a fractured tooth and the borders might be called the fracture line. But are the fine lines in the enamel on the labial surface fracture lines too?

Don't leave room for interpretation when submitting a claim to restore a fracture or crack. The fracture of a molar is the 10 mm mesial-buccal cusp and into the dentin.

Craze lines are normal features of flat surfaces of teeth that usually don't require treatment.

The fracture of the facial enamel of a central incisor isn't a craze line; it's a 5 mm × 10 mm sheared off enamel section on the mesial line angle creating a rough surface with the underlying dentin visible through the enamel shell.

17 Cracked tooth syndrome is composed of a group of signs and symptoms that may require treatment. Some clinicians may opt for full coverage for cracked tooth syndrome. The first key to claims submission is to thoroughly document the signs and symptoms that may not be readily visible on radiographs. Is the diagnosis justified? The second key is whether an alternate noninvasive treatment option was considered before an invasive treatment was rendered. The third key is whether there was a time period between initial diagnosis and a second visit to determine if the symptoms are occasional and episodic.

18 For claim resubmission, submit all of the original documents for benefit adjudication as if it is a new submission. Prepare as though a different reviewer will read the claim documentation. Don't assume that any of the previous documentation is retained. The new package must stand on its own merit. This is the right time to add additional information not submitted in the original package. Call out to the reviewer's attention the additional documentation that supports the claim.

Desktop procedures

Any process taken individually is easy to do. It's when individual processes are added together that it becomes difficult to do. To successfully execute multiple processes is exacerbated when they aren't linear or occur less frequently.

This is where desktop procedures become invaluable. Desktop procedures delineate what, when, and how to administer a dental claim. It's written and reviewed frequently. It's not done on an ad hoc basis nor is it the institutional knowledge of the most senior employee. It's not for the convenience of the staff but for the good of the business.

Write the desktop procedure using the guidelines in this chapter, revise at least annually, and monitor it frequently. The goal is to streamline the patient experience with no financial surprises. The goal is to maintain cash flow with little accounts receivable and bad debts. The goal is to get it right.

Conclusion

To get it right means fast, efficient, and effective dental claim submission that eases administrative headaches, increases cash flow, and creates a clear communication channel with the patient that increases rapport and trust.

To get it right isn't rocket science and doesn't require a business degree. It requires the dentist to establish the administrative system. The system starts with a clinical dental record that accurately reflects the diagnosis and treatment in as much detail as needed for any other reader to understand what occurred at that appointment. The clinical dental record is the patient's dental diary and not shorthand for billing. The dental record flows into the electronic financial system that allows proper submission of the dental claim from patient eligibility verification to payment from the patient and the third-party payer.

To understand the quirks in the system and follow the suggestions will stand the clinician in good stead. At the end of the day, the CDT Code is the reference that guides claims submission and the credo "bill for what you did" is sacrosanct.

PART II
Dental Claim System

CHAPTER 4

Patient-centered practice

David Okuji

NYU Lutheran Dental Medicine, Brooklyn, USA

Introduction

Imagine a crying and kicking preschool child being escorted back to a dental operatory for a dental filling and, against his wishes, the child's father is sternly instructed to wait in the reception area while the dental treatment is performed. Is this patient-centered care? A dentist practicing in 1980 would answer, "this is normal practice, and, yes, I am (underscore for emphasis) taking care of the patient." If you are a dentist practicing in the 21st century, you might respond, "No, this clearly is not patient-centered care," since 78% of parents choose to be present in the dental operatory with their children.

Indeed, in a generation's time, the dental profession has developed many elements of patient-centered care, which include the four principles:

1 Dignity and respect—A dentist should respect parental beliefs that their child's overall health is better if they are present in the treatment room for all procedure.

2 Information sharing—A dentist provides evidence-based information about the relative risks and benefits for parental presence in the treatment room.

3 Participation—A dentist provides the parents an opportunity to ask questions about parental presence in the treatment room and have the choice to make an informed decision.

4 Collaboration—A dentist supports a community and professional collaboration for leaders to meet and discuss the risks and benefits of parents in the treatment on the care of children.

These principles are important because the Affordable Care Act (ACA) bringing a new era of accountability, dentists need to practice patient-centered care to meet society's expectations of quality care.

Dental Benefits and Practice Management: A Guide for Successful Practices, First Edition.
Edited by Michael M. Okuji.
© 2016 John Wiley & Sons, Inc. Published 2016 by John Wiley & Sons, Inc.

Donald Berwick, former administrator of the Center for Medicare and Medicaid and founder of the Institute for Healthcare Improvement (IHI), offers three maxims on how to apply the principles of patient-centered care:

1 The needs of the patient come first.
2 Nothing about me without me.
3 Every patient is the only patient.

These maxims are important because in the future dentists may be rated by the level of service and care they provide to patients, much like hospitals are rated by the federal government-sponsored Hospital Consumer Assessment of Healthcare Providers and Systems (HCAHPS). Imagine if the government published an online rating service on all dentists that is made available to the public (Yelp on steroids). As well, these maxims translate the business principles of "customer service" to the world of health care—Think Nordstrom—where dentists must not only provide technical quality but must also provide the highest level of service quality.

However, even a 21st century dentist may balk at a parent's request that their dentist not apply fluoride to their child's teeth and not use restorative materials that contain silver amalgam or bisphenol A. So why should we, as dentists, follow the principles of patient-centered care? Don't we know what's best for the patient? Isn't that what we're paid to do? To answer these questions, this chapter delves into the idea that patient-centered care is a key component in transforming the health-care system; this transformation directly impacts dentistry and dentist who embrace patient-centered care will gain a competitive advantage in the marketplace. Fundamental change in the structure and process of the health-care system and delivering dental services is already taking place. Some examples of this change include the growth in the number of group dental practices and pay for performance based on quality and health outcomes. And as new health-care delivery models develop, patient-centered care will serve as the core strategy for competitive advantage. Those dental practices that do not adapt to this new market environment may not succeed and thrive in a field of forward-thinking competitors.

Key to transform the health-care system

The concept of patient-centered care emanates from the quality improvement movement that began in 1987 with the National Demonstration Project in Quality Improvement in Healthcare, founded by Berwick and A. Blanton Godfrey, former CEO of the Juran Institute. This project focused on the application of industrial quality improvement methods to the health-care industry, whereby 21 health-care organizations applied quality improvement methods learned from companies such as AT&T, Corning, Ford, Hewlett-Packard, IBM, and Xerox. In 1989, Berwick and other visionaries founded the IHI with a commitment to redesign "health care into a system without errors, waste, delay, and unsustainable costs" (Table 4.1).

Moving the agenda for health-care quality forward, the Institute of Medicine (IOM) published two seminal works. In 1999, *To Err is Human: Building a Safer*

Table 4.1 Principles to redesign health-care systems.

1	Healing relationship	Treat the whole patient not just the teeth
2	Customized	Treatment based on disease risk
3	Source of control	Respect for patient's belief system
4	Knowledge shared	Dentists are transparent
5	Evidence based	Share evidence-based knowledge
6	Safety	Patient safety is a system property and top priority
7	Transparency	Open to all pertinent stakeholders
8	Anticipate need	Anticipate future needs based on patient's unique clinical situation
9	Waste decreased	Continuous improvement to decrease waste and inefficiency
10	Cooperation	Interprofessional team with strong communication skill

Health System was published and concluded that tens of thousands of Americans die each year as a result of preventable mistakes in their care. The work laid out a comprehensive strategy by which government, health-care providers, industry, and consumers can reduce medical errors. Lives have been saved by applying quality improvement science, which has reduced medication errors, improved infection control practices, and decreased surgical procedures on the wrong site.

In 2001, the IOM next published *Crossing the Quality Chasm: A New Health System for the 21st Century*, which proposed a comprehensive national strategy and plan on how the health-care system could be reinvented to foster innovation and improve the delivery of care. Toward this goal, the committee presented a comprehensive strategy and action plan for the coming decade. Finally, in 2007, the IHI launched its Triple Aim initiative for populations. The Triple Aim applies and integrates approaches to simultaneously improve care, improve population health, and reduce cost per capita. The Triple Aim's motto is more simply stated as better care, better health, at lower cost.

With this in mind, we, as dentists, must join our medical colleagues and continue to innovate care delivery, which provides better care for our individual patients, better health for our community of patients, and care at lower cost. One example is the use of infant/toddler group dental visits whereby the dental office holds 1-h group visits with a group of 10 mother–child pairs. During the group visit, the dentist is able to provide in-depth educational information for the mothers, provide oral health assessments, and apply topical fluoride to the children's teeth. Thus, by seeing the mother–child pairs in a group, the dentist can meet the Triple Aim goals.

Crossing the Quality Chasm lays the foundation for patient-centered care on how to redesign and transform the health-care system. The key component related to patient-centered care outlines the six foundations for patient care rendered by a health-care system:

First, care must be safe and avoid injuries to patients from the care that is intended to help them (use of papoose board for combative pediatric patients for a short emergency procedure).

Second, care must be effective and provide services based on scientific knowledge to all who could benefit and refrains from providing services to those not likely to benefit (more frequent application of topical fluoride varnish for children at high risk for dental caries).

Third, care must be personalized (patient centered) and respectful of and responsive to individual patient preferences, needs, and values and ensures that patient values guide all clinical decisions (offer the use of composite resin material for patients who prefer not to be exposed to amalgam restorations, which contain mercury).

Fourth, care must be timely and reduce waits and sometime harmful delays for both those who receive and those who give care (respect patients' time and attend to patients at their scheduled appointment time).

Fifth, care must be efficient and avoid waste, including waste of equipment, supplies, ideas, and energy (share a CAD/CAM ceramic crown fabrication unit among dentists that practice independently in the same building).

Sixth, care must be equitable and provide care that does not vary in quality because of personal characteristics such as gender, ethnicity, geographic location, and socioeconomic status (caring for patients who are Medicaid beneficiaries at the same level as patients with commercial insurance).

The Triple Aim further specifies the primacy of patient-centered care and how it fits into the design of a health-care system. It is critical to note that this model illustrates how health-care quality is defined from the perspective of an individual member of a defined population and, thus, is a key component in transforming the health-care system. With the inclusion of pediatric dental services included in the ACA, the dentist must be cognizant of the Triple Aim objectives and its impact on how we provide care not only to our patients as individuals but also to our patients as a population.

Transformation: Impact on dentistry

Initiatives in the dental profession have lagged at least 15 years behind those same initiatives in medicine. Examples of the lag time between medicine and dentistry include the founding of the American Medical Association (AMA) and the American Dental Association (ADA) (15 years), establishment of the AMA and ADA code of ethics (19 years), creation of association-published professional journal (30 years), development of standards for specialty training (24 years), establishment of the American College of Surgeons and the American College of Dentists (7 years), formal recognition of health-care disparities (19 years), and leading quality improvement initiatives (22 years). Clearly, medicine is far ahead of dentistry with regard to developing structures, processes, and initiatives to support the health-care system.

The IOM outlines ten principles to redesign the health-care system. These principles include patient care that is based on continuous healing relationships care, which is customized to patient needs and values; care where the patient is the source of control; care where knowledge is shared and information flows freely; care where decisions are evidence based; care where safety is a system property; care where transparency is necessary; care where patient needs are anticipated; care where waste is continuously decreased; and care where cooperation among clinicians is a priority.

In addition, the IOM prescribed that the transformation of the health-care system's structure and process must be changed in four areas. The first principle is to apply evidence to health-care delivery. On average, it takes seventeen years for new, evidence-based knowledge to be incorporated into practice. The IOM recommends that private–public research partnerships be developed with a focus on priority conditions. An example is the National Dental Practice-Based Research Network (NDPBRN), which is a consortium of dental practices and organization with funding by the National Institutes of Health. The NDPBRN focuses on the efficiency and effectiveness of real-world dental practice. The second principle is the use of information technology, which has the potential to allow all stakeholders in the health-care system to communicate, analyze, improve the efficiency and effectiveness of health care, and eliminate the need for handwritten clinical data. As an example, dentists and medical providers could be connected through a health information exchange in order to share health information for mutually shared patients. Would it not be easier to confirm a dental patient's need for subacute bacterial endocarditis prophylaxis by accessing the patient's medical record by computer rather than playing telephone tag with the patient's cardiologist's office? The third principle is to align payment policies with quality improvement in order to eliminate perverse reimbursement incentives. A fee-for-service reimbursement system motivates dentists to perform more procedures with the potential for overutilization of services. A capitation reimbursement system motivates dentists to perform fewer procedures with the potential for underutilization of services. When the reimbursement system is aligned with quality health outcomes, the dentists are motivated to "do the right thing" for the benefit of the health of each individual patient and the population at large. Imagine a reimbursement system where a dentist is paid more to have 100% of patients under 4 years of age caries free rather than having 100% requiring full mouth rehabilitation under general anesthesia? The fourth and final principle is to prepare the workforce for success in the newly revamped health-care system created by the ACA. The workforce must be trained and learn to work harmoniously in interdisciplinary and interprofessional teams with the aim to provide patient-centered care that is safe, effective, timely, efficient, and equitable. An example is the previously described group appointment model whereby a dental hygienist or dental therapist is embedded in or colocated with a pediatric medical practice to conduct group appointments for mothers and their infants.

If you were to study the chronology and content of the IOM and IHI reports in greater detail, you would find that they serve as the underpinning for the 2010 ACA. The ACA contains all of the precepts espoused by the IOM and IHI with regard to patient-centered care. In addition, pediatric oral health care is one of ten essential health-care benefits in the ACA. Thus, federal law formally embeds the dental profession into the health-care system and opens the door for dentistry to integrate with the other health disciplines to transform health care by embracing the practice of patient-centered care and the Triple Aim: better care, better health, and lower cost. The greatest opportunity for integration is for dentists to participate in interprofessional health-care teams to improve the health of their mutual patients. What if a dentist is teamed with a diabetic care provider, provides updates on the patients' periodontal status, and serves as a health-care extender that monitors and reports oral and general health changes in the health information exchange network? Might the overall health of these diabetic patients be improved with coordinated communication and care by the team?

Clearly, through the IOM and IHI initiatives and the ACA, a sea change in the health-care system is taking place. More people now have health insurance, and a large number of these people are victims of health-care disparities due to low socioeconomic status. In addition, health-care providers must provide patient-centered care in an efficient and effective manner. Although dentistry has traditionally lagged behind medicine with quality of care and reimbursement initiatives, dentistry is now legally swept up in the rip tides, currents, and swells of the health-care system transformation. If medicine navigates these crashing waves on an aircraft carrier, dentistry is currently paddling in a dinghy. However, with the inclusion of dentistry in the ACA, dentists have the opportunity to get onboard medicine's aircraft carrier.

Transformation: Evidence in health care and dentistry

A large number of changes in the structure and process of the health-care system and dentistry are already taking place:
1 Two-tier financing system
2 Two-tier delivery system
3 Increased accountability expected by payers
4 Electronic health record
5 Integration of medicine and dentistry
6 Population health outcome
7 Emphasis on evidence-based care
8 Utilization of midlevel providers
9 Increase in the group practice model
10 Rise in the number of employed dentists

Two-tier financing
Both the medical and dental health-care systems participate in a two-tiered system of financing based on availability of financing coverage (Tables 4.2 and 4.3). According to *The Economist*, America is developing a two-tiered health system, one

Table 4.2 Medical financing by percent of US population (2012). http://kff.org/other/
state-indicator/total-population

Privately financed (%)		Publicly financed (%)			Uninsured (%)	Total (%)
53		31+			15	100
Employer (%)	Other private (%)	Medicaid (%)	Medicare (%)	Other public (%)		
48	5	16	14	1+		

Data from Kaiser Family Foundation. © 2015, Wiley.

Table 4.3 Dental financing by percent of US population (2004). http://meps.ahrq.
gov/mepsweb/data_files/publications/cb17/cb17.pdf

Privately financed (%)	Publicly financed (%)	Uninsured (%)	Total (%)
53.9	34.6	11.5	100

Data from Agency for Healthcare Research and Quality. © 2015, Wiley.

for those with private insurance, the other for the less well off. In 2012, medical care financing for the US population was comprised of 53% employer-sponsored health insurance programs, 32% government-sponsored programs such as the Medicare and Medicaid programs, and 15% without medical insurance coverage at all. In 2004, dental care financing for the US population was comprised of 53.9% privately sponsored programs, 11.5% government-sponsored programs such as Medicaid program, 34.6% without dental insurance coverage [1]. Therefore, in both medical and dental insurance coverage, over 53% of the US population is covered by privately sponsored insurance plans, which represent one tier of care, and the remaining 47% are either uninsured or covered by government-sponsored plans, which represent the second tier of care. This 47% of people in the second tier has less access to care since the uninsured tend not to seek health care and many providers, in particular dentists, do not accept patients with government-sponsored plans.

The financing of health care has undergone continual transformation in both medicine and dentistry. Typically, the government-financed Medicare reimbursement system institutes changes and then the government-sponsored Medicaid and commercial dental financing system follows. Examples of this lead and follow phenomena include:

1 The move from cost-based reimbursement system to a flat rate, resource-based relative value scale (RBRVS), prospective payment, diagnosis-related group system by Medicare in 1983 [2].

2 Health maintenance organizations that reimburse providers on a per-patient per-month basis in consideration for providing appropriate care for a panel of patients.

3 Preferred provider organizations that reimburse providers at a negotiated and discounted fee schedule.

Two-tier delivery system

Most medical and dental primary care is delivered by for-profit enterprises, such as solo practices and group practices. There is a variation in the delivery of medical and dental care to patients within a two-tiered financing system. Most medical providers render care to patients, regardless of the source of health-care financing. Specifically, most physicians accept patients with Medicare or Medicaid benefits. On a national level, more than 80% of physicians see new Medicare patients and 69% see new Medicaid patients. In contrast, most dentists do not accept patients who are Medicare or Medicaid beneficiaries. Only 10–25% of private practice dentists render care to a significant number of Medicaid patients. Dental providers don't sufficiently tend to the health-care needs of the second tier of patients because they are not sufficiently reimbursed to support their fragmented, inefficient dental delivery system.

Although most medical and dental primary care is delivered by for-profit enterprises, there is a large network of nonprofit federally qualified health centers (FQHC) that are chartered by the federal government to provide care to patients who are government-financed plan beneficiaries or are uninsured. FQHC include all organizations that receive grants under Section 330 of the Public Health Service Act and qualify for reimbursement from Medicare and Medicaid. FQHC must serve an underserved area or population, offer a sliding fee scale, provide comprehensive health services, establish an ongoing quality assurance program, and have a governing board of directors. Certain tribal organizations and FQHC look-alike meets PHS Section 330 eligibility requirements may receive special Medicare and Medicaid reimbursement but do not receive PHS grant funding. What is unique about the FQHC structure is that the majority colocate and integrate both medical and dental services. In 2011, 862 of 1128 (77%) FQHC integrated dental care as part of their scope of primary care services [3]. Therefore, the FQHC system serves as the primary care delivery system for the underserved population.

Accountability

Payers are increasingly holding providers accountable for the services rendered to the subscribers or beneficiaries of the payers. One prominent example is the government's use of recovery audit contractors (RAC) that are third-party contractors engaged by Medicare and Medicaid to identify and recover overpayments made to providers. Through a somewhat punitive process, the RAC is not specifically intended to identify fraud but instead is tasked to find improper Medicare and Medicaid payments. Hence, a dentist may be contacted by the state Medicaid RAC auditor and asked to reimburse the state for payments made for topical fluoride varnish procedures for children who are not at high risk for dental caries. Another example is the random quality assurance audit conducted by payers in order to ensure that providers are adhering to the terms and requirements of the participating provider agreement and provider manual. A more compelling example of accountability is the public posting of physician utilization and payment data for by Medicare [4]. According to a report by Bloomberg, which featured the Medicare posting, one ophthalmologist was paid $21 million by Medicare in 2012 [5].

Dentists are on notice that they are transparent and under the scrutiny of outside parties, particularly government payers, to be accountable.

Electronic health record

The Health Information Technology for Economic and Clinical Health Act (HITECH) of 2013 intends to improve the quality of care through the interoperable electronic exchange of health information based on the five pillars of health outcomes priorities:

1 Improve quality, safety, efficiency, and reduce health disparities
2 Engage patients and families in their health
3 Improve care coordination
4 Improve population and public health outcomes
5 Ensure adequate privacy and security protection for personal health information

Imagine a health-care world in which all providers can coordinate and communicate information about the care for their patients. Instead of communicating by paper, telephone, or fax, dentists can obtain consultations from cardiologists about the need for antibiotic prophylaxis for subacute bacterial endocarditis antibiotic prophylaxis through a secure network rather than waste time and resources through the use of the telephone or fax machine.

Population health outcomes

In a sophisticated HITECH world, patient data is deidentified, aggregated, compiled, and analyzed for population health outcomes. Note, however, that in order to analyze population health outcomes, dentistry needs to standardize and implement the use of diagnostic codes, as medicine does through the International Classification of Diseases (ICD-10). Currently, the dental profession only utilizes CDT procedure codes and does not use diagnostic codes. The three competing dental diagnostic code systems are the ADA-sponsored Systemized Nomenclature for Dentistry (SNODENT), the Consortium for Oral Health Related Informatics (COHRI) system called EZCodes, and the ICD-10 system. The SNODENT classification system has the objectives to:

1 Provide standardized terms to describe dental disease
2 Capture clinical detail and patient characteristics
3 Permit analysis of patient care services and outcomes
4 Be interoperable with Electronic Health Record and Electronic Dental Record

Health information technology serves as the backbone for information sharing as the ACA and the Triple Aim move forward improve health, improve the patient experience, and lower cost for the American population.

Integration of medicine and dentistry

This integration has taken root in a variety of ways. Examples of this integration include:

1 Association between oral health and general health—Research has demonstrated the association between periodontal disease and systemic diseases such as

preterm, low-birthweight newborns, heart disease, stroke, diabetes, respiratory infections, osteoporosis, and cancer [6].

2 Interprofessional education initiatives—In 2008, the Interprofessional Education Collaborative was established by the Association of American Medical Colleges, the American Association of Colleges of Osteopathic Medicine, the American Association of Critical-Care Nurses, the American Colleges of Pharmacy, the Association of Schools of Public Health, and the American Dental Education Association with the objective to develop a common set of competencies for interprofessional education and practice [7]. The Frontier Center at the University of Colorado, School of Dental Medicine serves as an interprofessional training center for medical, pharmacy, and physician's assistants to learn about oral health and dental students to understand systemic health. It supports a colocation project in which primary care students and dental students collaborate to provide interprofessional health care to special populations.

3 Clinical practice—The nation's FQHCs integrate oral and general health. Some health centers integrate a dental provider into the medical primary care or pediatric medicine department to provide oral health evaluations and preventive procedures in conjunction with the medical visit. One community pediatric medicine clinic integrates infant–toddler oral health education, evaluations, and topical fluoride applications with well-child visits in a group medical appointment format.

Population health outcome

One prong of the Triple Aim is "better health," which is measured through analysis of population health outcomes. The Medicare program changes the way it pays hospitals by paying for provision of high-quality services instead of by the number of services provided. The health morbidity of obesity can be used to illustrate how population health outcomes will be measured. The population health outcome is to increase the percentage of Americans with a healthy weight. Given this assumption and with an interoperable health information exchange, there are four areas of population health metrics that can be used to measure healthy weight. The first metric is to employ new technologies to integrate self-report with sensors, measure physical activity, diet/nutrition, and energy balance/obesity in real time. Exemplars are the technology of wearables such as the Fitbit and the Grush toothbrush that electronically monitor your child's tooth brushing technique. The second metric is to develop valid measures of community food access, food deserts, nutrition, and environments friendly to physical activity. Food deserts have been identified through the use of geographic information systems (GIS) technology. What if we integrated the use of wearable mobile sensors and GIS for community members who live in food deserts so we could determine where these individuals are actually obtaining their food and, in turn, measure their overall health metrics? The third metric is to integrate surveillance and other public or private information technology systems to monitor population body mass index, physical activity, food purchasing, and screen time (video games monitors). Again, wearable devices like the Fitbit are examples of how population health can be monitored. The fourth metric is to develop and implement national data standards for healthy weight/obesity, physical activity, and healthy food consumption across the life span. Standards for healthy weight can be developed when individual metrics are compiled into a national database.

Utilizing the population metrics for obesity as a model, dentistry could develop a model for the population outcomes to increase the percentage of caries-free children or to increase the percentage of adults without periodontal disease. What if we developed an electronic toothbrush with biometric sensors that not only measured the duration of brushing but also measured acidity, biofilm composition, and the buffering capacity of saliva. Data could be collected and analyzed for individuals so that dentists could provide prescriptive and therapeutic care. In addition, the data could be compiled on a national level in order to establish benchmarks for oral health.

Evidence-based care

In 2008, the Centers for Medicare and Medicaid Services proposed that the ADA assume the lead to establish the Dental Quality Alliance (DQA). The DQA develops performance measures for oral health and has the objectives to:

1 Identify and develop evidence-based oral health-care performance measures and measurement resources
2 Advance the effectiveness and scientific basis of clinical performance measurement and improvement
3 Foster and support professional accountability, transparency, and value in oral health care through the development, implementation, and evaluation of performance measurement

Current examples of the types of negative quality metrics considered by DQA include early tooth loss due to extraction or pulp therapy in primary anterior or molar teeth and restoration within 24 months of application of sealants on permanent molar teeth. Like fresh cement, the foundation to develop population health metrics and outcomes has been laid, and as the foundation cures, medical and dental professionals need to understand how to improve population health through evidence-based care. The Cochrane Collaboration defines evidence-based health care as the conscientious use of current best evidence in making decisions about the care of individual patients or the delivery of health services. Current best evidence is up-to-date information from relevant and valid research about the effects of different forms of health care, the potential harm from exposure to particular agents, the accuracy of diagnostic tests, and the predictive power of prognostic factors. The Choosing Wisely campaign, sponsored by the American Board of Internal Medicine Foundation, has moved to translate the use of evidence-based medicine into clinical application by creating lists of medical tests and procedures that providers and patients should question. It is interesting to note that currently no dental specialty group is represented on the Choosing Wisely list.

In comparison, the Image Gently campaign includes the dental profession and spotlights a set of succinct recommendations to help protect children from radiation exposure through unnecessary radiographs. These examples are opportunities for the dental profession to join the medical profession in translating evidence-based dentistry to clinical application.

Midlevel provider

Clayton Christensen, the Harvard Business School professor renowned for his theory on disruptive innovation, applied his disruption innovation theory to the health-care industry. The key idea for disruptive innovation in health care is that less skilled practitioners can manage more complex procedures than they currently provide. In Christensen's disruptive innovation model, he uses the example of nurse practitioners. The nurse practitioner is capable of treating many medical problems that used to require a physician's care. It is highly probable that the last time you went to the physician's office, you were seen and treated by a midlevel provider or another physician extender who examined you and wrote a prescription for your ailment.

The dental profession is undergoing a similar disruption with the advent of dental health aide therapists who are licensed to provide unsupervised dental procedures in Alaska, Minnesota, and Maine. Disruptive innovation will continue in the health-care arena through the use of midlevel providers. With the use of midlevel dental providers such as dental therapists, access to care may be expanded to underserved populations. As well, for-profit dental practices may leverage the use of midlevel providers in order to treat more patients at lower cost since the compensation level of a midlevel provider should be far less than that of a dentist. An owner of a dental practice would most likely prefer to employ a lower paid dental therapist to manage simple procedures rather than employ a highly paid dentist.

Group practice model

In both the practice of medicine and dentistry, more practitioners are becoming employees of institutions such as hospitals and group practices. The move for hospitals to buy doctors' practices has been growing steadily in the past decade as care increasingly shifted from inpatient hospital care to an outpatient setting. In the 10 years between 2001 and 2011, the number of physicians and dentists employed by hospitals across the USA grew by more than 40%. The ADA Health Policy Institute indicates the number of dental office sites controlled by multiunit dental companies increased by 49% to 8442 locations from 1992 to 2007. As the practice of dentistry evolves from a solo sport to a team sport, younger dentists will prefer to work as employees for dental groups because they can practice dentistry without the burden of operating a business, forego spending money for a dental office, enjoy family time and lead a balanced life, pay off educational debt rather than add to their debt load, work on a part-time basis, gain clinical experience, enhance their skills, and enjoy the collegiality and tutoring of experienced dentists. In short, younger dentists can concentrate on delivering care and earn a good income without the burden of starting and managing a practice. As in medical care, the delivery of dental services trends toward aggregation with a rise in the numbers of group practices and dentist employees. It is clear that dental and medical practice is undergoing a dramatic transformation in the structure, process, and outcomes of the health-care system. These changes impact the financing system, accountability of providers to payers, delivery system, electronic health record, integration of dentistry and medicine, population health outcome, evidence-based care, use of midlevel providers, and practice employment models. It is incumbent upon dentists to become fluent in all of these aspects of the transformation so they can effectively compete on the basis of patient-centered care.

Oral health-care delivery model

Prior to describing new health-care delivery models, let's examine the nature of organizational structures with their respective strengths and weaknesses. By understanding the typology of organizational structures, a dentist can determine how to integrate patient-centered care within the structure. First described are the five basic organizational types that include process, functional, divisional, matrix, and network structures. This examination of structure typology is followed by a discussion on network organizations since the new models for health-care delivery are based on the network structure.

Organizational structure

Process form organizational structure focuses on the linear process of taking inputs, processing the material, and generating an output. An example of a process form organization is a solo dentist's practice that accepts patients into the office, renders care, and completes care for the patients, who return for periodic recare visits.

The functional form organizational structure is designed for centrally coordinated specialization. The key term is that a functional form is centrally coordinated with the budget and directives managed centrally by management. An example of a functional form health-care organization is a stand-alone group practice that is organized by specialty departments such as general dentistry, dental hygiene, pediatric dentistry, endodontics, periodontics, and oral surgery that are centrally controlled by executive management.

Divisional form organizational structure creates divisions that are autonomous and serve their respective markets. The divisions are subject to a centrally controlled performance evaluation and resource allocation. An example of a divisional form health-care organization is a geographically distributed practice model that has multiple small group practices located across a region. Each practice is free to serve its local market and has its performance monitored and resources allocated by the executive management.

Matrix form organization is based upon a functional form, which is centrally controlled from the top and overlays a horizontal cross-management team to serve special markets. An example of a matrix form health-care organization is a functional form small group practice, as described previously, which serves a commercially insured population and now wishes to create a fee-based loyalty program for high-income patients who desire no waiting time for appointments and concierge dentistry. This practice would have a concierge, or case manager, who is responsible to ensure that loyalty program patients obtain readily available and convenient appointments and receive concierge care. The concierge coordinates with each functional group (general dentistry, dental hygiene, endodontics) so that the loyalty patients receive the proper care.

Finally, as network forms move from a structure of vertical integration and instead, disaggregates the organization by developing alliances with independent suppliers and distributors. Although it is a marketing firm and not a health-care delivery organization, an example of a network form organization is 1-800-Dentist, whose members pay a subscription fee for collective marketing services.

Network organizations share the following traits: (i) they use collective assets of several firms along the value chain (Toyota leverages the established business relationships of suppliers and subsuppliers to obtain low prices and high-quality supplies for its chain of suppliers); (ii) they rely more on market mechanisms than administrative processes to manage resource flows (Toyota's suppliers keep track of Toyota's supply inventory rather than Toyota internally managing this function); (iii) they expect a proactive role among network participants in order to improve the final product or service (Toyota's suppliers must ensure that it supplies high-quality supplies and service so that Toyota is successful and will retain the suppliers in the network); and (iv) they exhibit cooperative and mutual shareholding (Toyota executives sit on the board of directors of many of its suppliers) [8].

There are three types of network organizations: stable, internal, and dynamic. A stable network has the operating logic of the functional form where a core firm serves a predictable market by linking together independently owned specialized assets along the value chain. As example of a stable health-care network is Pacific Dental Services (PDS) based in Irvine, California. PDS provides management services for its geographically distributed network of dentists who own their respective dental facilities. An internal network utilizes commonly owned business elements allocate resources along the value chain using market mechanisms. An example of an internal network is Coast Dental and Orthodontics, which privately owns over 180 offices throughout the Southwestern and Southeastern USA. The dynamic network links independent business elements along the value chain form temporary alliances from among a large pool of potential partners. An example of a dynamic network is a state-wide independent practice association (IPA), which links a large number of small, independent private practices.

Organizational structure: Opportunity

With the disruptive transformation of the health-care system come opportunities for new delivery models and competitive strategies for dental practices. As previously described, the dental group practice model is fast becoming the preferred delivery model for dental services due to the economies of scale and the preference of younger dentists to work for a larger firm. The ADA classifies dental group practices into six categories: (i) integrated medical and dental practice, (ii) networked and integrated medical/dental practice, (iii) stand-alone or networked large group practice, and (iv) the networked solo dental practice.

Integrated medical and dental practice

This practice model would look very much like the FQHC that is previously described and is allocated in one patient catchment area. The advantage of this model is that it fully integrates medical and dental practices for the benefit and convenience of its patients. The patient care is coordinated in a one-stop shopping experience with presumably better health outcomes. For-profit entities could emulate this model whereby a group of dentists, either in group practice or solo practice, would affiliate with a group of primary care physicians to establish a system of medical and dental providers to serve a local patient catchment area. As an example, in a small farming town of 40,000, a small group general dental practice and a small primary care medical practice partner together to provide integrated care for its pool of patients. The patients receive integrated care with the dentists and physicians with data shared via an electronic health exchange. The integrated group gains a competitive advantage over its solo practice competitors. In another example, assume a city with a population of 100,000 and a large group dental practice and a large primary care medical group that integrate care for its pool of patients. In this example, patients receive integrated care with shared data through a centralized electronic health record. This large integrated group gains a competitive advantage over its local competitors and has, to some degree, leverage in negotiating reimbursement levels from payers because the integrated group can guarantee to payers a menu of services that fragmented providers cannot guarantee. As a specific example on the Monterey Peninsula of California, with a population of 105,242, the Monterey Peninsula Dental Group might partner with the Ryan Ranch Medical Group to establish a medical–dental integrated group. The integrated dental–medical entity can offer 6 day a week office hours, a full range of dental specialist care, pediatric hospital care, 24-h dental emergency care, and, even, dental offices with colocated nurse practitioner screenings for the dentist's medical counterparts. This practice model resembles the networking of two internal network organizations.

Networked and integrated medical/dental practice

This practice geographically expands the patient catchment area and provides care to a larger region. This model is similar to the example above with the integration of dental and medical group practices but expands the model to multiple local, state, or multistate geographic regions. With an interoperable health information system, the networked and integrated practice shares patient data across a large geographic area. In addition, the large networked and integrated practice benefits from economies of scale, which is one key in reining in the cost of care. Far beyond a purchasing cooperative, these arrangements allow for population health through colocation and shared health information and a far better mechanism for recruiting, training, calibrating, mentoring, nurturing staff, HIPAA and OSHA compliance, credentialing system, clinical care oversight, and clinical outcome measurement compared to what a smaller operation can offer. For example, the Hawaii Family Dental Centers group could partner with the primary care physicians of Hawaii Permanente Medical Group to serve the entire 1.4 million population of Hawaii. Both groups have geographically distributed offices on the four major islands of Hawaii and an array of services that fits an accountable care organization. This practice model is a prime example of an integrated dental–medical network of two stable network organizations.

Stand-alone networked large group dental practice

This practice models currently exist and geographically expand the patient catchment area by providing care to a very large population. Examples of a stand-alone large group practice include Heartland Dental Group, Coast Dental and Orthodontics, Gentle Dental, and Bright Now! Dental. Although the stand-alone networked large group delivers care to wide geographic regions. But imagine if just two of these groups strategically merged into one coordinated super group. This is similar to airline mergers that consolidate market share and take advantage of the economies of scale. This practice model has the characteristics of a network comprised of multiple stable network organizations.

A networked solo practice

This model can be established on a local, regional, or national level through the establishment of an IPA model. In 2004, there were 163,447 working (133,690 general and 29,757 specialist) in private practice. An IPA model incorporates the following characteristics: (i) practice ownership retained by each provider, (ii) broadly shared financial risk when contracting for participation in health plan networks that allows a degree of collective bargaining, and (iii) a defensive strategy against managed care plan. The key element is that the IPA can function as one entity to represent the mutual interests of the IPA member dentists. Imagine if the 163,447 dentists who practiced independently in 2004 established a regional or national IPA. An IPA model opens the possibility for the independent solo dental practitioner to consolidate information technology, employee training, and human resource recruitment, training, and retention expertise into one entity that streamlines a practice. This practice model exemplifies a dynamic network organization.

The adage, necessity is the mother of invention, applies to dentists in the era of the ACA and the Triple Aim. The transformation of the American health-care system necessitates that dentists become innovative to design and implement new models to deliver care, which is aligned with the Triple Aim initiative.

Patient-centered care: Competitive advantage

The topic of patient-centered care is revisited and described as a competitive advantage for those who can master its practice. Recall that patient-centered care is the key driver for the Triple Aim enterprise that defines quality from the perspective of an individual member of a defined population. Each individual member is a customer who needs to receive a valued service and utility from their experience in the health-care delivery system. If the patient–customer is not pleased with the value and quality of the care they receive, they look to competitors for future services. Worse yet, the consumer may tell family members, friends, and colleagues not to patronize the practice. Therefore, it is critical that dentists become experts in delivering patient-centered care, regardless of the delivery model. In health care, this value to the patient and the health-care system is determined in the equation $VALUE = QUALITY \div COST$ where value is driven by higher quality, lower cost, or both.

Michael Porter, Harvard Business School competitive strategy guru, illustrates that patient satisfaction is a key element in the valuation equation [9]. The Division of Hospital Medicine at the University of California, San Francisco, includes patient satisfaction as one of three major components for quality in the value equation and specifies HCAHPS score and patient complaint as metrics for patient satisfaction [10]. Digging deeper into what constitutes patient-centered care, the IHI lists twelve domains that patients and families expect for patient centeredness from health-care providers:

1 Are we listened to, taken seriously, and respected as care partners?
2 Have my family/caregivers been treated the same?
3 Do we participate in decision making at the level we choose?
4 Are we always told the truth?
5 Are things explained to us fully and clearly?
6 Do we receive an explanation and apology if things go wrong?
7 Is information communicated to all my care team?
8 Is care timely and impeccably documented?
9 Are records made available to us if requested?
10 Is there coordination among all members of the health-care team across settings?
11 Are we supported emotionally as well as physically?
12 Do we receive high-quality, safe care?

These twelve qualities are simple to understand, and it is imperative that providers of care and leaders of health-care organizations pay full attention to the consumer. When dentists don't practice with a focus on patient-centered care, they are at risk to fail when consumers and payers do not value their services.

The Commonwealth Fund goes further and lists six key attributes of patient-centered care that provides a framework on how to practice patient-centered care on a daily basis:

First, dentists must provide education and shared knowledge (evidence-based information is shared with patient and family).

Second, dentists must include the involvement of family and friends (family and friends are encouraged to be involved with the care of the patient).

Third, dentists must practice collaboration and team management (provider team has strong communication and team skills).

Fourth, dentists must exhibit sensitivity to the nonmedical and spiritual dimensions of care (patient's cultural and spiritual beliefs are respected).

Fifth, dentists must have respect for patient needs and preferences (overall respect for the patient's belief system).

Sixth, dentists must deliver the free flow and accessibility of information transparency of health information.

Let's compare the custom of care between 1980 and today by applying the six attributes of patient-centered care to the previously described example of the small child whose father was instructed not to accompany the child into the dental treatment operatory, despite the father's expression of desire to accompany his child (Table 4.4).

With the social evolution of parenting practices between 1980 and the 21st century, parents are more involved in the care and supervision of their children and are less trusting of authority figures who are involved with the care of their children. Clearly with this example, most pediatric dentists have adapted to the change in parenting styles and have made improvements in developing the capability of rendering patient-centered care. However, we, as a profession, have a long way to go in order to inculcate the practice of patient-centered care within the domain of oral health. Many dentists still make patients wait for their scheduled appointments, do not provide convenient hours of operation, and do not provide clear explanations of the cost and description of planned treatment.

Table 4.4 Attributes of patient-centered care.

	1979	2014
Was the father provided education and shared knowledge?	No	Yes
Was the father involved in the care?	No	Yes
Was there collaboration and team management?	No	Yes
Was there sensitivity to nonmedical and spiritual dimensions of care?	No	Yes
Was there respect for the father's needs and preference?	No	Yes
Was there a free flow of information?	No	Yes

The Commonwealth Fund further delineates seven key factors that contribute to patient-centered care on the organizational level:

1 Leadership, at the level of the CEO and board of directors, sufficiently committed and engaged to unify and sustain the organization in a common mission (dentist owner and board of directors must maintain a strong commitment to patient-centered care as a strategic advantage).

2 Strategic vision clearly and constantly communicated to every member of the organization (dentist owner must communicate the patient-centered care vision to all staff members and "walk the walk").

3 Involvement of patients and families at multiple levels, not only in the care process, but also as full participants in key committees throughout the organization (patients, parents, and caregivers are valuable stakeholders, and their views and perspectives should be heard as it pertains to the quality of patient care).

4 Care for the caregivers through a supportive work environment that engages employees in all aspects of process design and treats them with the same dignity and respect that they are expected to show patients and families (nonfamily member caregivers must be given the same respect as the patient and family members as they are integral in the care of the patient).

5 Systematic measurement and feedback to continuously monitor the impact of specific interventions and change strategies (measurement through quality improvement science methods should be used to monitor and evaluate changes in process interventions).

6 Quality of the built environment that provides a supportive and nurturing physical space and design for patients, families, and employees alike (physical space of the practice should be conducive for supportive and nurturing patient care).

7 Supportive technology that engages patients and families directly in the process of care by facilitating information access and communication with their caregivers (dentist owner should invest in technology that provides convenience, accessibility, and transparency for patient care communication).

It is these organizational challenges on which we must focus to achieve success in providing patient-centered care. Health-care organizations that master these structural elements of patient-centered care gain a significant competitive advantage over organizations that are unable to do so. If an organization is unable to support the critical element of patient-centered care, it will be at great risk of failure since patients and payers may not value the organization.

Conclusion

Dentists must develop a strong patient–customer focus in order to remain competitive in the health-care arena. It's not a matter of feel good public relations for the financially fat dental practice but a fundamental matter of survival.

Failure to embrace the patient-centered credo dooms any practice model that does address the marketplace that values patient-centered care. Dental group practices, especially large multisite dental entities, face marginalization when they adopt a dentist-centric private practice strategy and merely put it on steroids. Dental organizations are wise to consider the legendary Nordstrom model of customer service in which the customer is the primary focus. Jamie Nordstrom, the great-grandson of founder John Nordstrom, says, "customer service is things that customers value over and above the product they buy," and goes on to say, "the cornerstone of the business has always been the people and we spend a lot of time talking about how we can improve our team.... It's the topic at most of our meetings" [11].

Health-care organizations become successful when they focus on customer service (patient-centered care), develop its team of people (create a supportive work environment and provide training), and invest in information technology for measurement, feedback, and quality improvement. The 21st-century dentist must focus on customer service and patient-centered care in order to be competitive and economically successful in the era of the ACA and the Triple Aim. Long gone are the days when a dentist's office is only open 4 days per week so the dentist can play golf. It is clear that the focus has shifted the importance of health care toward the health of the patient, health of the population, at lower per capita cost. Dentists who achieve these objectives will be rewarded and thrive, and those who don't will be irrelevant.

References

1 Medical Expenditure Panel Survey 2007 Dental Use, Expenses, Dental Coverage, and Changes, 1996 and 2004. http://meps.ahrq.gov/mepsweb/data_files/publications/cb17/cb17.pdf (accessed August 6, 2014).

2 Office of the Inspector General. 2001 Medicare Hospital Prospective Payment System: How DRG Rates are Calculated and Updated. https://oig.hhs.gov/oei/reports/oei-09-00-00200.pdf (accessed August 29, 2014).

3 Hilton IV. Interdisciplinary collaboration: What private practice can learn from the health center experience. *Journal of the California Dental Association* 2014; 42 (1): 29.

4 Centers for Medicare and Medicaid Services. Medicare Provider Utilization and Payment Data: Physician and Other Provider. http://www.cms.gov/Research-Statistics-Data-and-Systems/Statistics-Trends-and-Reports/Medicare-Provider-Charge-Data/Physician-and-Other-Supplier.html (accessed December 20, 2014).

5 Bloomberg.com. 2014 Top Medicare Doctor paid $21 million, Data Show. http://www.bloomberg.com/news/2014-04-09/top-medicare-doctor-paid-21-million-in-2012-data-shows.html (accessed December 20, 2014).

6 Cullinan MP, Ford PJ, Seymour GJ. Periodontal disease and systemic health: Current status. *Australian Dental Journal* 2009; 54 (Supplement 1): S62–S69.

7 Valachovic RW. Integrating oral and overall health care – On the road to interprofessional education and practice: Building a foundation for interprofessional education and practice. *Journal of the California Dental Association* 2014; 42 (1): 26.

8 Miles RE, and Snow CC. Causes of failure in network organizations. *California Management Review* (Summer 1992): 53–72. http://www.uniovedo.es/egarcia/milesysnow.pdf (accessed September 23, 2014).

9 Porter ME. What is value in health care? *New England Journal of Medicine* 2010; 363: 2477–2481.

10 The Healthcare Blog. 2013 *How UCSF is Solving the Quality, Cost, and Value Equation.* http://thehealthcareblog.com/blog/2013/05/27/how-ucsf-is-solving-the-quality-cost-and-value-equation (accessed September 21, 2014).

11 Apparel. 2012 Nordstrom's Big Secret Revealed. http://apparel.edgl.com/case-studies/Nordstrom-s-Big-Secret-Revealed-82375 (accessed September 25, 2014).

CHAPTER 5

Streamlined dental practice

Michael M. Okuji[1] & Dennis Lewis[2]

[1] *Delta Dental of Colorado, Denver, USA*
[2] *Dental Aid, Inc., Louisville Colorado, USA*

Introduction

Change or become irrelevant. Change or perish. The current route to small practice model that is so favored by dentists is to borrow funds, choose a location, equip with high technology, staff, and the 4-day workweek. Then it's on to earn enough revenue to support these style choices. It's all about the dentist's chosen lifestyle. The chosen style is clearly not patient centered and financially unsupportable to the point of perpetual angst it creates that focuses on the need for higher fees for an increased number of procedures to a constant flow of new patients.

While we may think that all dentists fit under the revenue bell curve, what we see is a bimodal distribution of dental revenue among dentists. So, the dentists on the left peak are stressed to either move to the right (produce more revenue) or streamline the practice (lower operating cost) to achieve comparable income.

To streamline a competitive dental practice is to implement the processes critical to deliver patient-centered care. Going forward, it's not about the dentist and it's all about the patient. The consumer, the customer, and your patient will have access to information to make them discerning consumers of dental services. The competitive landscape for dental care delivery will focus on access, health outcome, and cost of care. Those dental practices that consistently deliver on the Triple Aim will attract more customers, more patients.

To make a change when we're comfortable in what we do is counterintuitive. To make a change when everyone around us stays the course seems foolhardy. But to make a change when we can't pay the rent next week is just too late. The road to financial failure occurs in small almost imperceptible increments.

So, let's first take the short-term view to streamline practice processes that are baby steps, easy, and inexpensive. After that, let's look streamline practice processes that are long term, take time to implement, take a personal commitment, take a financial commitment, and take a leap of faith. It's okay to not be the innovator, early adopter, or even in the early majority when it comes to

Dental Benefits and Practice Management: A Guide for Successful Practices, First Edition.
Edited by Michael M. Okuji.
© 2016 John Wiley & Sons, Inc. Published 2016 by John Wiley & Sons, Inc.

streamlining your office. But to be in the late majority or a laggard to streamline practice processes is a decision that is fatal to the dental enterprise.

To streamline your practice in the short term means to first take the easy baby steps. Take the baby steps today and don't wait for tomorrow. Baby steps prod you to think in terms of administrative (process) management. Baby steps are entirely in your control; change the things you can change.

Begin to implement processes that efficiently capture and deliver information and improve cash flow—a dollar today is worth more than a dollar tomorrow. The baby steps are electronic processes to determine dental benefit eligibility, predetermination of treatment, insurance claim submission, and direct deposit. These steps break through the major administrative bottleneck that impedes the start of treatment and increased cash flow. The baby step captures accurate information internally and then disseminates it externally to the payer and the patient. This is streamlined and patient-centered care in one single process.

Chapter 5 walks you through steps to identify the streamline points in a practice, define outcome measure, and the infrastructure necessary to deliver services in a streamlined practice.

Private practice

We're all familiar with the solo dental practice, where the dentist hangs their shingle in a location of their choice, in an office of their design, equipped to their specifications, and operated to suit their needs that often mean office hours that end at 5:00 on a 4-day week. The practice operation is designed to match the dentist's vision of their ideal world; build it and they will come. To streamline this practice model means to not only implement administrative systems to make the operation run smoothly but to also to implement the systems that make the operation patient centered.

Systems and operation

You're encouraged to think in systems and not ad hoc situations. Ad hoc thinking is for a particular purpose, whether that is charting, radiographs, treatment planning, dental records, financial bookkeeping, insurance claim submission, or appointments. Systems or operational thinking takes the whole process and rationalizes them to achieve system efficiency and patient satisfaction. Let's walk through the dental practice administrative system from the first encounter to the money in the bank.

Electronic eligibility

Patients are generally unaware of the details of their dental benefits. It is not unreasonable for you to expect the patient to take responsibility to know and understand their dental benefit before they come to you. There are numerous benefit companies—some with offices in different states and multiple plan designs with different waiting periods, maximums, and limitations. There are too many dental benefit permutations for any dental office to intimately understand. In reality, patients probably don't know much beyond the name of the benefit company. But when you think about it, how much do you know about your medical benefit coverage when you see your physician? Do you know the waiting period, deductible, limitation, frequency, coinsurance, and copayment for the medical procedure you are experiencing?

So, to check patient eligibility and benefits is the first baby step. But never ever do it by telephone communication. Telephone transactions take too much administrative time, can lead to miscommunication, and don't archive the transaction. Check patient eligibility electronically through the benefit company's website or interactive voice response (IVR) system. This is a free service web portal. Third-party vendors like OneMind Health® bundle this service with other services for you for a fee.

Predetermination

The electronic process begins with the predetermination of benefits. Treatment predetermination is a critical administrative and shouldn't be overlooked. You should predetermine a case where a financial misstatement will cause significant patient dissatisfaction, for example, increasing an orthodontic truth-in-lending agreement after treatment has commenced and the first payment is made. Electronic predetermination is fast and efficient. Costs vary for the service depending on the attachment requirement. For some third-party payers, there is no cost when you utilize their secure web portal. A rule of thumb is to predetermine a benefit if you would be unhappy to write off the procedure fee. For instance, would you predetermine a $125 prophylaxis? Would you predetermine a $1500 ceramic crown? Most will say no to the former and yes to the latter, and this makes sense because a benefit payment error that results in zero reimbursement is less detrimental to the patient ill will in the former than the latter. Predetermination of root canal or a crown makes sense because they are big-ticket items that result in a significant patient portion. Predetermine big-ticket items. There must be no second-guessing.

For many procedures, a predetermination of a benefit is not reviewed by a person and is adjudicated by the computer in seconds. The computer algorithm looks for patient eligibility, wait period, plan design, frequency of service, limitations, history, and then applies the deductible, allowance, and patient portion. All of this occurs on the day of service within seconds of receipt because you didn't send it via US Mail. To just start the process, it wasn't necessary to open an envelope, sort the paper claim, input the claim into the system, adjudicate, print the report, enter into a queue, and then return to you via US Mail. Attachments should be submitted only if requested by the benefit carrier and then only as an electronic attachment. Radiographs, periodontal charts, and narratives can all be sent electronically. If you submit a crown for predetermination today, you would have it in hand before the patient presents for the treatment.

Dental software supports electronic predetermination and electronic attachments. There is a cost for these third-party services, but the cost is less than paper submission by your staff and less than the cost incurred to print and post. Some dental benefit companies support electronic predetermination and electronic attachments through their web portal at no cost to the provider.

The benefit for the dentist, dental office, and patient to electronically file a predetermination is not inconsequential. A predetermined claim makes the benefit amount and patient amount for the procedure clear and unambiguous. A predetermined claim eliminates any financial misunderstanding between the dentist and the patient. Clear and accurate information is a critical feature of a dental practice that is patient centered and streamlined.

Claim submission

To submit a dental claim, be promptly paid, and collect the patient balance take an inordinate amount of time. It takes a substantial amount of time to train and supervise the dental claim administrator. Inevitable benefit error costs the practice money and time. A benefit error costs the practice substantial good will and trust with the patient. So, to process a claim efficiently and accurately is a challenge and total cost to administer the dental claim process is not inconsequential.

This is where electronic predetermination and claim submission are essential and the most effective. One key to benefits administration streamlining is to key an entry once and only once. After the treatment note is keyed into the electronic dental record (EDR), the clinical information should flow to the predetermination, claim submission, claim adjudication, claim reconciliation, and claim payment.

Electronic claim submission

Once the treatment information is keyed for the predetermination information, there is no need to rekey it again all the way through the payment of the claim. Electronic filing of a predetermination means no rekey, no printing, no stamp, and no waiting for the US Mail to deliver and return. It takes a few seconds to enter the date of service on the predetermination and submit it electronically. The administrative time and cost saving from electronic services are not inconsequential. In a predetermined case, the patient portion is accurately collected and the benefit payment credited to your account overnight. Your accounts receivable turnaround time and accounts receivable aging are zero. Any past problem to collect the patient portion balance long after the case is complete is a problem of the past: happy patient, happy dentist, and happy office.

Electronic direct deposit

A dentist who doesn't care whether they get their money as fast as possible is making too much money to care. General Motors understands that a dollar today is worth more than the same dollar tomorrow. There is no reason to wait for your money because of a mailed claim, paper printing and batching, check printing, and return mail. Even a clean paper claim can take weeks to process.

The benefit company can help set up a direct deposit account. All it takes to register a direct deposit account is a bank account number and bank routing number. Both of these numbers are on the bottom of every paper check you write. Some dentists are reticent to register their bank information with a benefit company for direct deposit because of a fear of security. But all of the information needed to open a direct deposit account is readily available on every check you write.

Check reconciliation is done either through an electronic alert or through the benefit company's web portal. Every step of electronic reconciliation is the same as with a paper check stub only faster. A direct deposit accounts a lifeline to maintain cash flow in the case of a natural disaster when all mail service is curtailed. In Colorado, when towns hit by winter storms and torrential spring floods are shut down for weeks, US Mail delivery ceases and paper check stops arriving, while electronic deposits continue to be deposited.

To have your money quickly available for your use is a primary tenant of all businesses. Cash flow and cash control are key to business viability. Money on the books, your accounts receivable, only counts when it's in your bank account. The longer money is left on the books, the less valuable it becomes and the more difficult it is to collect.

The turnaround time between when the service is performed and when the fees are in your bank should be minimized. The combination use of electronic predetermination, claim submission, and direct deposit shortens or eliminates the dental payment and patient accounts receivable turnaround time. Patient portion balances disappear and the accounts receivable account goes to zero when the patient portion is collected upon the predetermination of benefit. A dentist who thinks that having a bank balance sufficient to pay monthly bills is the indicator of a healthy cash flow is either not fully aware of the time value of money or is just making too much money to care.

EDR

The next steps are long-term projects that require more commitment, time, and money from the dental practice to successfully incorporate. The EDR allows you to collect the various parts of the patient record into a single cohesive document. It is more than a tool to compile financial records, bill claims, and print statements. The EDR tells a story; the story is about your relationship with the patient. It tells the reader the presenting issue, pain, and recare; patient concern; assessment of the health history; assembled records; diagnosis; treatment plan; prognosis; follow-up; and next thoughts. It is the patient's health record.

The EDR is so clear and complete that the patient or another dentist can ascertain why, what, when, how, and who did the treatment without ambiguity. How much detail needs to be entered into the EDR? As much or little as to tell the story without the reader having to guess. We know that most restorative procedures require local anesthesia; maybe you use the same anesthetic with the same vasoconstrictor in the same amount on every restorative case. But the record must tell the reader what, where, and how much anesthetic is administered in every case. You know and the reader must know too. We know that you standardize the steps to surgically extract an erupted tooth. But the EDR must tell the reader the steps you took: flap opened, bone removed, tooth sectioned and elevated, and sutures to close to make the story clear.

The EDR is standardized for every patient and every patient encounter so that critical information isn't overlooked. For instance, the ideal dental record prompts a dentist to query if osteomyelitis is noted on the health history prior to implant body placement. The EDR is not a set of shorthand notes to jog the dentist's memory nor is it a document designed just to submit a dental claim.

The EDR in the near future includes the ability to share dental information between dental offices and share medical information between health-care providers. The streamlined EDR in the near future includes diagnosis codes linked to a procedure code in order to track patterns of practices and outcomes. The EDR of the near future integrates with the patient's medical records so that their physician can route to you the pregnant patient for dental care or the child in need of anticipatory guidance, the dentist can route to the physician the patient out of sync with diabetic medication, high blood pressure trends, and obesity and anorexia medical issues.

There is no excuse to be in the paper chart world. To store patient charts, radiographs, financial records, and old insurance claims in your garage is an unacceptable way to manage a streamlined practice. Electronic bridges between dental software and medical software, like the EPIC medical record system, are being built today. The EDR is a requirement for a dental practice to deliver on the promise of a streamlined and patient-centered care.

One shortcoming of the current EDR system is that it is built for an exclusively dental platform. EDR systems, which are principally a financial administrative program, are written in a silo that doesn't interact with other EDR systems or medical record systems like EPIC. This means that dental information can't be shared between proprietary systems and historical information is lost when a patient transfers to a different provider.

This EDR shortcoming is overcome when an information technology integrator rationalizes the dental delivery system around the dental galaxy model and regional group practice systems (Chapter 9). The consumer benefits from this type of streamlined dental galaxy because of the easy portability of their EDR, medical–dental record integration, multiple points of access to care, and outcome driven care.

Access to the dental record

The streamlined, patient-centered dental office of the near future allows patient's access to their dental record an easy and accessible feature of their practice. This means that a patient can enter and update their personal information online. This means that a patient can access online their personal diagnosis, treatment plan, prognosis, and treatment progress. This means that a patient can access online benefit coverage, financial record, and schedule an appointment anytime, anywhere.

For example, Kaiser Permanente members view their health record, communicate with their provider, schedule an appointment, and see their statement anytime online. When they move between facilities and providers, their health records are available to everyone in the system. Kiosks in the facility allow them to check in and pay a bill. Members of the Kaiser Permanente system expect this level of streamlined service and will, in the future, expect this streamlined kind of service from their dental provider too or find another dental provider that offers the service.

Access to the personal dental record is a major step to be accountable and transparent. Aspects of the Affordable Care Act on and off the insurance exchange will further drive accountable and transparent practices. The transparent personal dental record reveals the diagnosis, treatment, outcome, and fee associated with a particular episode of care. Patients will be able to compare and contrast their dental care with the community.

Perhaps of greater importance is that the current systems don't support dental–medical integration. This means that important information generated from a dental encounter like elevated blood pressure, weight gain, behavioral concern like anorexia, change in medical history, current dental finding of medical concern like punched out bone in a radiograph and positive Bence-Jones protein, and adherence to current prescription regimen like cardiac and diabetic regimens is not readily transferred to the medical provider or simply lost in the transfer and follow-up. In medical encounters, caries incidence in children, untreated periodontal disease that exacerbates multiple medical issues, and pregnant women without a dental encounter are lost opportunities for dental intervention at the appropriate time.

An integrated medical–dental record is an essential link to deliver patient-centered care both in the dental and medical realm. An integrated health system like Kaiser Permanente that combines financing, hospital, medical care, and outcomes is the most likely integrator of the medical–dental health record. The medical–dental link can provide Kaiser Permanente physicians with additional sources of important patient information that is more significant to them than the annual physical examination like blood pressure trends. The newly formed Institute for Oral and System Health at the Marshfield Clinic Research Foundation in Wisconsin promises to tackle the integration of medical and dental care, clinical support systems to improve the quality of patient care, and lower overall health-care costs.

Diagnostic code

In addition to being limited as a dental-only record, another shortcoming to the current EDR system is that it is built to capture only procedure codes, that is, what individual procedure is rendered so that a dental claim can be filled and submitted for payment. Procedure codes that are captured in the EDR are the American Dental Association Current Dental Terminology (CDT) code set that is used by third-party payers to adjudicate dental claims for payment. What it doesn't capture is the diagnosis; why the procedure was performed. Dentists write into their dental record and submit dental claims on what they did but are weak or silent on why they did the procedure. The reason a diagnostic code set is important and relevant is that they underpin the understanding of practice patterns that lead to certain health-care outcomes.

This shortcoming may be addressed in the near future by integration into the EDR diagnosis codes captured in ICD-10, SNODENT, and EZCode code sets that become the standard for the industry. In anticipation of dental diagnosis codes, Box 34 and 34a on the ADA Dental Claim Form J430D is a placeholder to enter diagnosis codes when they become mandatory. Matching the diagnosis code to the treatment code takes dentistry a long way down the path to finally address patterns of practice that are tied to better health outcomes.

Airline analytics

Dental practices have administrative roadblocks in their system that decrease efficiency and increase costs. The broken and missed appointment is one such roadblock that leaves a fully staffed facility idle. This is one system issue that can be addressed with analytics borrowed from another industry. The airline industry attacks the issue and never lets a plane fly half full nor lets a plane fly with potential paying passengers left at the gate. Airlines use data analytics for modeling that predicts capacity needs. Unlike a dental practice, an airline doesn't blindly overbook a set number of passengers on every flight every day.

Dentists collect troves of clinical and nonclinical data on their patients and never use it to improve service, raise revenue, and control cost. Dentists have access to years of appointment books, demographic information, procedures delivered, benefit coverage, and payment history. In the instance of chronic broken appointments, the standard advice is to educate patients about the value of dental care or simply double or triple book their appointment. Both solutions are inadequate and nonsensical. To try to change behavior is a challenge and to double book is a haphazard management. A better solution is a predictive model that takes into account the multiple variables that surround a broken appointment. Examples of broken appointment variables are seasonality, day of the month, time of day, patient satisfaction (how well they were treated clinically, administratively, personally), type of procedure, and method of payment. For a community health clinic that treats primarily children, to book middle school-aged children during the week of school district-wide testing is folly. This is just one simple example of predictive analytics that doesn't require rocket science to improve a process in a streamlined practice.

Airlines lead other industries in the application of operations research and information technology to develop predictive models to tackle the problem of optimal capacity and productivity. To understand how airlines quantify productivity goes a long way to address how to streamline the dental practice. Besides the broken appointment, other productivity issues for dental practice process improvement include empty chairs in the underutilized facility and staff allocation. Airline companies face the same optimization and productivity challenges with empty seats, expensive equipment, highly trained and costly crew, and lost revenue opportunity once the plane leaves the ground. The airline must operate fully crewed safe equipment whether the plane has one passenger or is at capacity. The airline also doesn't want to leave too many passengers at the gate that will go to a competitor. As far as seat capacity and other metrics, the dental practice is no different and can benefit from aggressive data mining and data analytics. Airlines analyze multiple ratios that include load factor, airline seat miles, revenue per mile, revenue per available seat mile, and cost per available seat mile. Each of these metrics has a counterpart in dental practice.

One reason dentists often cite for not wanting to treat patients covered by Medicaid is that they are more likely to miss appointments. The citation is an impression not supported by investigation and can be a self-fulfilling prophecy that justifies not treating Medicaid patients. The Sarrell Dental Center (Alabama) reports that it achieves over 95% seat occupancy when it applied operations analytics to historic patient data and aggressively utilized its call center. The Sarrell Dental Center is an example of aggressive data mining and data analytics to successfully address an important operations problem.

Sarrell Dental Center

The Sarrell Dental Center (Sarrell) is a community health center in Alabama that grew from 1 clinical site in 2002 to 14 clinical sites in 2014. During this period, its operating revenue grew from less than 1 million dollars to over 16 million dollars without any grants and gifts. The Sarrell Dental Center revenue and revenue growth outstripped three Colorado dental care community health centers (Figure 5.1). It's earnings before interest, taxes, depreciation, and amortization (EBITDA) are 9% where other community health centers would run a deficit if it were not for grants

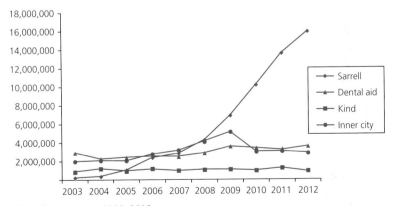

Figure 5.1 Clinic revenue 2003–2012.

and gifts that make up 40% of their operating revenue. Sarrell Dental Center is often cited as an innovative dental care model not because it is clinically superior but because it is a superior business model. The Sarrell business model is illustrative of a streamlined system that can be adopted by small practice, dental group, and dental group system. The business model is competitive because of how it views the customer. For Sarrell, it's about service to their customer who is a patient. Sarrell streamlines its operation with the customer in mind. For instance, Sarrell offices are open 6 days a week and stay open until the last patient is seen.

Call center

Taking another best practice from the airline industry, the Sarrell Dental Center business model uses a dedicated call center staff. The call center staff's primary responsibility is to maximize the chair utilization. They use their existing patient database to make reminder telephone calls and reschedule missed appointments. When the parent of a child chooses to use Sarrell, the call center staff schedules an appointment at a time and location most convenient for the parent. Sarrell's locations offer extended office hours, which include evenings and Saturdays, to better accommodate a family's schedule. At Sarrell, it's all about the patient and not about the dentist.

Data analytics enables call center staff to book the number of appointments that results in targeted treatments, minimized patient wait times, and avoids excessive patient load for clinical staff. Optimal chair utilization is critical to maintain consistent facility utilization, optimal revenue, and spread expense over a wide footprint to maximize the net income. The cost and effort to streamline the practice are more than worth the financial investment.

Call center staff track and monitor individual patient show rates on a daily, weekly, and monthly basis that feed into the database and analytic tool. Getting seats filled is such a fundamentally critical feature of productivity that call center staff are among the better paid members of the Sarrell team and receive performance-based incentives.

Administration

Sarrell Dental Center streamlines its operations in other areas too. Sarrell supports a dedicated billing department with extensive experience with Medicaid and Children's Health Insurance Program (CHIP). Claims are processed quickly without error that result in a consistent cash flow that supports the operations and company growth. Sarrell streamlines to cross-train staff members so they perform multiple roles in each office according to need. Many call center staff members are cross-trained to be dental assistants and front desk staff.

Workforce

The efficient and effective business model relies on a dedicated, motivated, and talented workforce. To keep the talent, Sarrell offers growth opportunity in its system and pays for vocational, graduate, and dental school education for its staff.

Beyond that career progression, Sarrell offers staff members a compelling vision of purpose to its young staff, to do something positive for the society and to help all children to access the dental care and the habits that stand them in good stead for a lifetime. It promotes a culture of caring.

Community

Sarrell doesn't wait for the patient to walk into the door. Each office has a community outreach coordinator who works with county and local community organizations, day care facilities, and schools to organize free, basic dental screenings. The community outreach coordinator offers oral health education to children and parents at health fairs, PTA meetings, and classroom visits. Sarrell sponsors and conducts community outreach activities like a program that brought Santa Claus to communities to take free pictures with the kids and free summer sports camps for kids with Sarrell-branded giveaways. The community outreach programs provide the opportunity to increase Sarrell's visibility and provide opportunities to recruit children who do not currently have a dentist or dental provider.

Medical–dental integration

Beyond dental treatment, Sarrell takes the encounter opportunity to streamline and improve medical–dental integration. At each appointment, the child's height, weight, blood pressure, and temperature are taken, and a copy of this information is given to each parent. Sarrell instituted this data collection and dispersion as standard practice because many of the children do not see a primary care medical provider on a regular basis. If the child is overweight or obese, one-to-one oral health education is provided during the visit that is tailored to provide information about the importance of healthy eating and physical activity. Children are referred to their primary care giver if they have an elevated temperature or high blood pressure. Parents, other family members, and caregivers are encouraged to be present in the room during the exam. The oral health team takes this time to explain the importance of good oral health habits and provide a detailed explanation of any dental problems the child may have. Treatment recommendations are discussed with both parent and child.

Sarrell Dental Center team

Sarrell, with 14 clinical sites, has over 210 employees that include a clinical team that consists of 51 full-time and part-time dentists, 41 full-time dental hygienists, and 18 dental assistants. Dentists are not assigned to a clinic; instead, they work in different clinics on a daily basis. As a result, a dentist is not assigned to a specific group of patients. However, to ensure continuity of care, extensive notes are recorded in their EDR that each provider reviews before the patient's appointment. This method also allows many trained dentists to review recommended treatment plans and ensure optimized care is delivered to the patient. Sarrell's leadership points to the program's active cultivation of a "culture of caring" as a reason why its system of rotating providers works. According to program leadership, this "culture of caring" is operationalized in multiple ways, including the clinic décor, expanded hours of operation, reminder phone calls, follow-up calls to inquire as to why an appointment has been missed, requesting that the parent to be present in the room while the child receives care, the one-on-one education for parent and child during the exam, and extensive community outreach efforts.

Quality

It seems that in dental practice quality is in the eyes of the beholder. In a world where dentists work in a small private practice with no daily interaction with other practitioners, the view of quality is more "I know when we see it" and the application of quality is more "what I decide to do at the time I do it." We apply quality to matters large and small but mainly limited to technical process like "Are my crown margins closed?" Dentists focus on technical measures as a proxy for quality. But treatment patterns vary significantly between dentists where some procedures of known value like sealants are under used, treatments that are unnecessary and inefficacious are performed regularly, and treatments of dubious value like the Sargenti endodontic technique are embraced. Dentists treat the cost of care as immaterial, and you either provide high-quality care to a particular patient or you do not.

Quality has multiple attributes and the Institute of Medicine of the National Academy of Sciences defines quality as "the degree to which health services for individuals and populations increase the likelihood of desired health outcomes and are consistent with current professional knowledge." The Agency for Healthcare Research and Quality defines quality health care as "to do the right thing, at the right time, in the right way, for the right person, and have the best results possible."

Quality to the consumer may be different. Consumers may focus on how long they wait for an appointment or how much discomfort they experience from the treatment. From their perspective, health-care quality means to get the right treatment at the right time, in the right amount, with the right outcome, at the right price. The consumer, your patient, needs information to make a decision regarding their care to determine how well the dental care system meets their needs.

So, as we move forward to streamline the dental practice, the dentist needs to embrace quality metrics that keeps a focus on evidence-based care that is embedded in the profession's body of knowledge that tracks patterns of practice that lead to better health outcomes. In a preventive practice, this can mean the frequency of fluoride applications or the number of sealants that leads to less incidence of dental disease. The Dental Quality Alliance of the American Dental Association has developed performance measures for oral health care that can be tracked within each practice to determine whether "quality" care is delivered.

The streamlined practice that incorporates quality measurement is well prepared to compete for patients in the new normal that is dentistry. This means that a practice should transmit their demonstrable (accountable) and clear (transparent) quality metrics to the public. The benchmark pattern of practice with positive outcomes is the kind of information that health-care exchanges and benefit companies will require of its professional providers and individuals will access to choose their dentist.

Social determinant of health

Dental care delivery doesn't occur in a vacuum but rather as a part of the larger community. To streamline a practice means more than just the mechanical processes to run a business. The dental provider acts and interacts with patients from backgrounds and cultures other than their own. Social determinants of health are conditions that circumscribe the population that we want to serve. They need to be understood to streamline the practice and frame our competitive strategies.

Social determinants of health are conditions of the environment in which people live, learn, play, and work that can affect the health. The individual's available resources influence their quality of life and health outcomes. A few examples of these resources include safe housing, access to education, available healthy food, dependable transportation, language, literacy, and access to affordable health care. Dentists should be sensitive to how social determinants contribute to their patient's ability to accept the treatment plan, complete the recommended treatment, and the behavioral change needed to maintain good oral health.

Healthy People 2020, the US Department of Health and Human Services 10-year goals for health promotion and disease prevention, highlights five key social determinants of health. Health and health care is one of the five general areas. Access to health care, specifically access to affordable oral health care, must be considered by dental providers at both the organization and individual practitioner level for oral health to be considered as part of an integral to overall health. Oral health providers will be asked more and more how we intend to meet the needs of the uninsured, the publically insured, those with a primary language other than English, and people who simply were never taught the importance of disease prevention and the maintenance of good oral health.

In order to meet the needs of the entire spectrum of our community, we must reconsider such practices as dismissal of a patient every time they are 15 min late to an appointment. The patient could be a single mother of four who made a long bus trip with a connection to get her child to the dental office. The social determinants that lead up to her late arrival should be considered before she is dismissed. It may be a long time before this woman considers another dental visit if she must be reappointed. Her children's oral health only worsens during this delay. In short, to understand the social determinants of health allows us a framework to treat everyone with compassion for the individual and what they are dealing with in their lives that is different from our lives. It allows us to better meet our patients where they are and establish ways to get them healthier. One dental plan in Arkansas reimburses travel expenses to certain patients. An Alabama network of dental offices don't close until every patient is served.

Patient support system: Case management

A case manager assists a patient through difficulties and anticipates potential barriers to navigate our health-care system and receive the care they need. Our health-care system is a daunting and a complicated road to navigate. Imagine that English is your second language and you must navigate the health-care system blind and mute. You experience a kidney problem that demands a consultation with a specialist practicing at a large metropolitan hospital. The hospital has clear and ample signage to help you find your intended destination for your appointment. The problem for you is that the signage and direction arrows use the word "nephrology" and you are simply lost.

A case manager answers questions for their patients to assist them to understand the signs. In dental care, they assist them to understand the importance of oral health. Do they know they should visit a dentist during pregnancy and that it is safe? Do they know children should see a dentist close to the child's first birthday? Like a social worker, the case manager assists their patient to negotiate applications to obtain insurance for which they are eligible like health insurance subsidized through the Affordable Care Act and federal support from Medicaid. The case manager answers patient questions about treatment, medication instructions, and postoperative care. The case manager understands the social determinants of health their clients are facing then lowers the hurdles and helps remove the barriers to access care. Through case management, fewer appointments are missed, instructions are better understood, and health outcomes are improved. Case management establishes a deeper level of relationship than a dental care provider can reach in a 1 h visit where the treatment is the primary focus. As the oral health-care system expands, case management is one way to streamline the dental practice and improve both short- and long-term health outcomes.

Disease management

In dental school, we are very well educated and trained. We know the science behind decay. We know what to eat and how to brush and floss to prevent decay. In addition, we spend endless hours and are extremely well trained on how to restore the damage done by the dental disease.

But we are not well educated and trained to assess a patient's risk for dental disease, how to intervene very early in a child's life, and how the oral health of a child's family could influence their oral health. We graduate from dental school exquisitely trained to treat the symptoms of dental disease but not to manage or prevent the disease. If the disease dentist treated were polio, we would have the best iron lungs in the world.

Oral health providers treat the chronic diseases caries and periodontal disease. Dental disease is of epidemic proportions in many pediatric populations. In dental disease management, we should consider our goal as to prevent and control dental disease. Individual dental care plans should include periodic examination, preventive treatment, and periodontal maintenance frequencies assigned according to risk, not familiarity. Annual bitewing radiographs and semiannual prophylaxis for everyone are not a plan but rote formula. Some patients may require semiannual visits, while others require biennial visits. The individual care plan includes diet recommendation and home care regimen assigned according to risk. An informed patient can be actively engaged and control rather than just accept treatment for their oral health, a case of teach a man to fish.

To understand the social determinants of health is to improve oral health, not just treat dental disease, through our understanding of the environment and culture in which our patients live and thrive. Through the utilization of a case manager to actively engage and guide patients to take ownership of their health and disease management that focuses on risk, prevention, and maintenance, we streamline the dental practice and streamline the health-care system to achieve the goal of better health outcome.

Generational determinant of health

We can try to segment the population to design streamlined practices whether we try to hit all segments or target specific population segments.

Generation Z has never been without technology and expect communication. Gen Zs expect communication in short, informative bites. They expect text appointment confirmation, Yelp like review to select a service, and quick efficient service. Gen Zs are quick to change dentists.

Generation Ys, millennials, are technology dependent, want instant gratification, hate waiting, and do not expect to work for one company all their lives. The streamlined practice provides the option for additional services at each visit, combines appointments, and invests in the technology that offers same day service.

Generation Xs are high achievers that focus on good dental health for appearance and buy into the concept of whole body health care.

Baby boomers define respect for their dentist. Baby boomers prefer to be talked to in person or by telephone. They are raised on one-to-one transactions. Baby boomers often have resources to pay for treatment. They do not have dental insurance. Take the time to explain their treatment.

When looking at the generations of consumers, it's useful to look at the upcoming trends to visualize the future. For instance, a practice with a lot of baby boomers may be vibrant with patients today but dwindles with each passing year with no like-minded replacements in view. On the other hand, a new practice that treats children can expect yearly patient growth as the full effect of the ACA and consumer choice takes hold.

Conclusion

To streamline a practice is to improve the administrative process, increase the patient-centered experience, and be competitive. It's not a cosmetic makeover or a feel good experience. After taking the first baby steps, the streamlined practice uses the power of data and metric analysis to raise the quality and lower the cost of care. The Sarrell Dental Center is an example of a successful business model that harnesses the power of predictive data analytics.

A streamlined practice incorporates quality measurement, analysis, and implementation and understands the social determinants of health. Both of these are patient centered with a laser focus on the patient experience and healthy outcomes to treat a diverse community in a manner in which they wish to receive care.

Streamlining is the price a small private practice, group practice, group dental system, or community health center pays to become a productive, profitable, and sustainable player in the dental care delivery system. A streamlined practice is competitive and the dominant player in any segment it chooses to serve.

CHAPTER 6

Patient Protection and Affordable Care Act

Michael M. Okuji[1] & David Okuji[2]
[1] *Delta Dental of Colorado, Denver, USA*
[2] *NYU Lutheran Dental Medicine, Brooklyn, USA*

Introduction

The Patient Protection and Affordable Care Act (ACA) signed into law on March 23, 2010, stands as the most important piece of health-care legislation since President Johnson signed Medicare into law in 1965. Americans have not seen anything like the ACA given size, scope, and power of the federal government. The ACA and the Health Care and Education Reconciliation Act of 2010 sweeps up every American and expands Medicaid coverage and makes improvements to both the Medicaid and Children's Health Insurance Program (CHIP). Together, they promise that everyone will acquire health insurance that is administered and delivered in the private sector.

Some key provisions of the ACA are guaranteed coverage that requires health insurers to issue policies to any eligible applicant without regard to health status, community rating where the health insurer evaluates the risk factors of the market population and not the risk factor of any single individual, the individual mandate where all individuals are required to carry health insurance or pay a penalty, federal health insurance subsidies for individuals and families with incomes between 100 and 400% of the federal poverty level (FPL), and a health insurance purchasing marketplace for the individual and small business to purchase their health insurance.

The secretary of the Department of Health and Human Services has authority over commercial individual and employer-based health insurance. The ACA insurance provisions contain certain mandates for individuals, employers, insurers, and providers of health care that are enforced by the Internal Revenue Service with tax penalties. The constitutionality of the individual mandate to purchase health insurance has been upheld by the Supreme Court as a tax, although states are not required to participate in Medicaid expansion. Under the ACA, providers

Dental Benefits and Practice Management: A Guide for Successful Practices, First Edition.
Edited by Michael M. Okuji.
© 2016 John Wiley & Sons, Inc. Published 2016 by John Wiley & Sons, Inc.

are required to comply with federal standards for health plans and quality reporting, case management, care coordination, best practices, evidence-based care, and health information technology.

ACA quality

In addition to just financing health care, the ACA seeks to improve the quality and efficiency of health-care services for everyone with the payment for service linked to better quality outcome. It seeks to inform the consumer about health outcomes that result from different treatment choices and care delivery models.

The ACA establishes a national strategy to improve health-care delivery, improve patient health outcomes, and improve population health. It encourages strategies to develop, test, and expand innovative delivery and payment models including accountable care organizations that take responsibility for the cost and quality of care and receive a share of the savings derived from lower cost of care with better outcomes. The ACA authorizes the development of new programs and benefits related to the preventive services of school-based health clinics and oral health-care prevention education campaigns.

The ACA supports the enhancement of workforce training programs for general, pediatric, and public health dentistry, alternative dental health-care providers, and a US Public Health Sciences Track for dentists, physicians, nurses, and nurse practitioners.

The ACA's vision goes far beyond the financing of health care. It encompasses how individuals purchase and measure the process and outcome of health-care delivery and the health-care workforce. Further, accountable care and transparency of care as it pertains to the providers of the care are game-changing elements with ramifications to all health-care providers including dental care providers.

Health-care insurance marketplace

The key feature of the ACA is the requirement that all US citizens must purchase health insurance. The ACA seeks to increase the affordability of health insurance and reduce the cost of health care to individuals. It provides for a health insurance marketplace where consumers are given information to make informed choices on their health-care insurance.

Public exchange

The federal health-care insurance marketplace, the exchange, serves individuals or the Small Business Health Options Program (SHOP) for small businesses. Consumers without health insurance can purchase health insurance through the public health insurance marketplace. Consumers shopping for health insurance are those who never had insurance, lost their employer-sponsored plan, are prior individual purchasers, or are in transition from Medicaid. Businesses with less than 50 employees can purchase their health insurance on the SHOP Exchange.

Table 6.1 Health-care insurance marketplace by state and the District of Columbia.

Federal facilitated (15)	Federal with state plan management (7)	Federal individual with state SHOP (1)	State sponsor (14)	State–federal (7)	State on federal website (3)
Alabama	Kansas	Utah	California	Arkansas	Nevada
Alaska	Maine		Colorado	Delaware	New Mexico
Arizona	Montana		Connecticut	Illinois	Oregon
Florida	Nebraska		District of	Iowa	
Georgia	Ohio		Columbia	Michigan	
Indiana	South Dakota		Hawaii	New Hampshire	
Louisiana	Virginia		Idaho	West Virginia	
Mississippi			Kentucky		
Missouri			Maryland		
New Jersey			Massachusetts		
North Carolina			Minnesota		
North Dakota			New York		
Oklahoma			Rhode Island		
Pennsylvania			Vermont		
South Carolina			Washington		

As a small business, dentists in private practice can purchase health insurance for their office staff, their family, and themselves through the exchange. Effective in 2017, the states may allow large employers to purchase health insurance through the SHOP Exchange. The public health-care insurance marketplaces (the exchange) are either a federally facilitated exchange, a state-sponsored exchange, a state–federal partnership, or a state using the federal exchange website (Table 6.1).

Private exchange

Private health insurance exchanges are an emerging player in health insurance products. It's another option for employers to provide health insurance to their active employees and retirees. Rather than the employer selecting the health insurance benefit for their employee, the employee selects their own health plan from the offerings on the private exchange. Employees can select the insurance plan that best meets their needs. Employers find this attractive because the private exchange facilitates the migration of health insurance benefits to a defined contribution plan that caps their cost rather than a defined benefit plan. In a defined contribution plan, the employer provides a set dollar amount toward health coverage, and the employees use that money toward the purchase of health insurance from the insurance carriers on the exchange their employer has selected. Private exchanges cater to employer groups rather than individuals and small groups on the public exchange. Private exchanges tend to be flexible and can tailor a plan to meet the need of an employer group.

Private exchanges rely on sophisticated software platforms that take the shopping experience for insurance products to a new level. In many ways, it replaces the employers' human resource department with a consumer approach that directly involves the user of the product. The four general types of group sponsor private exchanges are insurance company exchanges, like the Cigna exchange, designed to protect their market share; a broker exchange, like the Aon Hewitt exchange, designed to keep the insurance broker and consultant relevant as employers migrate their employees to exchanges; technology company exchanges, like Swift, which started as outsourced benefit administrators and now provide infrastructure; and new technology exchanges, like Liazon, which provide flexible, technology systems. The American Dental Association and its state associations now direct members to a health insurance exchange for insurance products.

ACA

Ten sections (titles) comprise the Patient Protection and ACA [1]. As the ACA continues to mature, some sections will endure, some will be modified, and some will be deleted [2]. While there will be modifications and revisions, it's not expected that the ACA will be completely repealed.

Title I: Quality, affordable health care for all Americans

This section lays out the fundamental transformation of health insurance in the United States through shared responsibility of all its citizens, government, and the private sector. Systematic insurance market reform eliminates discriminatory practices like the individual preexisting condition exclusion and community rating. This means that individuals can't be denied insurance coverage because of a preexisting condition and their premium price is determined by community experience and not the individual experience. To achieve these goals means that everyone must be part of the system and must have health-care coverage. Individuals between 133 and 400% of the FPL receive a subsidy. The FPL for 2015 is $11,770 for one person.

Title II: Role of public programs

This section strives to improve access to Medicaid and expands the program to lower income levels and enhances the CHIP. This section also provides for the development of the medical care home concept that moves consumers from episodic care to a team-based care approach.

Title III: Improve quality and efficiency of health care

This section is of considerable importance to dentists. Many of its provisions may change the way dentists view dental care delivery. This section provides substantial investment to improve the quality and delivery of care to transform the health-care delivery system. It addresses the move from the fee-for-service system toward payments based on quality and cost efficiency. Part 2, Section 3013, refers to quality measurement development, and Section 3014 refers to quality measurement. Title III addresses changes to related public health law in Section 399JJ, "Public Reporting of Performance Information," by saying that the secretary shall make available to the public certain performance information on quality measures. This is a significant issue for dentists who practice in the world of experience-based care and procedure codes rather than evidence-based care and diagnostic codes. The proposed changes will start in the Medicare and Medicaid segment and then is expected to migrate to the private sector. Part 3, Section 1115A, refers to the Center for Medicare and Medicaid Innovation testing models of care delivery that include patient-centered, medical home models; transition of primary care practice away from fee-for-service-based reimbursement toward comprehensive or salary-based payment; contracting directly with providers of services to promote innovative like risk-based payment; and promote care coordination between providers of service. Part 3, Section 3022, Medicare Shared Savings Program," amends the Social Security Act to provide for the formation of accountable care organizations.

Title IV: Prevention of chronic disease and improve population health

This section addresses chronic illness and provides the infrastructure to improve population health. Subtitle A, Section 4102, speaks to oral health-care prevention activities.

Title V: Health-care workforce

This section addresses innovation in training, recruitment, and retention of the workforce. Subtitle C, Section 5203, refers to health-care workforce loan repayment programs, and Section 5207 refers to funding for National Health Service Corps. Subtitle D, Section 5303, refers to training in general, pediatric, and public health dentistry and provides financial assistance to dental students, residents, and practicing dentists. Section 5304 refers to alternative dental health-care providers' demonstration project grant for fifteen entities in the amount of no less than $4,000,000.

Title VI: Transparency and program integrity

This section is to provide information to the public so they can make informed decisions and a robust program to eliminate fraud, waste, and abuse in the delivery of health care. Subtitle D, Section 6301, refers to patient-centered outcome research.

Title VII: Improve access to innovative medical therapies

This section is primarily to improve access to generic drugs with biologics price competition and innovation.

Title VIII: Community living assistance service and support

This section fosters national voluntary insurance programs to purchase community living assistance services and support. It creates a system similar to the current Social Security disability system.

Title IX: Revenue offset provision

This section lays out how to pay for the elements of the ACA. Subtitle A, Section 9001, introduces an excise tax on high-cost employer-sponsored health coverage, and Section 9010 imposes an annual fee on health insurance companies including dental insurance companies.

Title X: Strengthen quality, affordable health care

This section addresses (i) the definition and implementation of a quality strategy and public reporting; (ii) a national strategy for quality improvement in health; (iii) the development of outcome measures for providers with clinical practice guidelines; (iv) the selection of quality and efficiency measures; and (v) data collection and public reporting. The section addresses the development of quality measures, collecting quality data, analyzing the data, and reporting the results. Quality of care reports will be unblinded and outward facing to the public. Quality is not in the eye of the beholder. The ACA is serious about the quality of health care and dentistry should be too.

Key provisions

There are a number of key ACA provisions that address equity and access to health-care insurance. The key provisions are guaranteed issue, community rating, and the individual mandate. These key provisions address adverse selection that undermines pricing by including the entire population into the risk pool. Guaranteed issue means coverage for all eligible applicants, ends the preexisting condition exclusion, and prohibits rate setting based on health status, medical condition, claims experience, and other factors. Community rating means that premiums vary only by family structure, geography, actuarial value, tobacco use, and participation in a health promotion program and the insurer evaluates the risk factors of market population and not those of any one person when premiums are calculated. The individual mandate means everyone is obligated to purchase health insurance or pay a penalty. Health insurance exchanges, both public and private, establish a health benefit marketplace in which the individual and small business can purchase health insurance. Individuals and families below 133% of the FPL are eligible for expanded Medicaid coverage. Individuals and families from 133 up to 400% of the FPL receive a federal subsidy to purchase health insurance. All health insurance plans have minimum standards with no annual and lifetime maximum. Firms with more than 50 employees that do not offer health insurance have a shared responsibility requirement if their employees receive a government health-care subsidy.

This all-in design for individuals and families provision levels the playing field for the consumer to purchase health insurance. The missing element to the ACA is an all-in design for provider provision, where all providers are obligated to accept the offered health insurance.

ACA essential health benefits

Every health insurance plan sold on the exchange offers 10 essential benefits:
1 Pediatric services including dental and vision care
2 Outpatient care (ambulatory care)
3 Emergency service
4 Inpatient care (care in the hospital)
5 Pregnancy, maternal, and newborn care
6 Mental health and substance use disorder services including counseling and psychotherapy
7 Prescription drugs
8 Rehabilitative services to help with injury, disability, or chronic condition
9 Laboratory services
10 Preventive and wellness services and chronic disease management

The Department of Health and Human Services deferred the decision of the essential health benefits (EHB) to each state. A state may benchmark its EHB from the three largest small group plans, three largest state employee plans, three largest federal employee plans, and the largest HMO plan. In every instance, pediatric dental services must be offered to everyone on the health-care exchange but is not required to be purchased by anyone.

Medicaid expansion

Medicaid expansion through the Health Care and Education Reconciliation Act of 2010 promises significant changes to both Medicaid and the CHIP [3]. Coverage for newly eligible adults is fully funded by the federal government for 3 years beginning 2014 and extends CHIP authorization through 2019 and CHIP funding through 2015. Additional federal funds for state Medicaid programs are available for primary care, preventive care, and new demonstrations to improve quality and reengineer delivery systems. Medicaid expansion seeks to improve the quality of care and the manner in which care is delivered and to reduce costs, essentially the Triple Aim. To increase Medicaid program integrity, Medicaid expansion includes provisions to terminate providers who have been terminated from other programs, suspend Medicaid payments based on credible allegations of fraud, and prevent inappropriate claims payment.

ACA funding

The Congressional Budget Office determined that the ACA would cover more than 94% of the population and stay within the $900 billion limit set by the president. This reduces the deficit over the next 10 years and bends the health-care cost curve downward. The Congressional Budget Office forecasts that the ACA's $604 billion in health-care expenditures will be offset by net receipts of $813 billion that results in a $210 billion reduction in the deficit for the 2012–2021 period.

A number of fees and taxes fund the ACA. The Medicare payroll tax rate increases by 0.9% (that's part of your payroll tax deduction), and an unearned income tax for high-income taxpayers is 3.8%. Health insurance companies pay an annual fee ($60 billion) as do pharmaceutical manufacturers and importers. There are an excise tax of 40% on "Cadillac" health plans ($32 billion), an excise tax on medical device manufacturers, a 2.3% tax on medical device ($20 billion), and an annual fee assessed on manufacturers and importers of branded drugs ($27 billion).

Drivers of health-care reform

The United States spends more of its gross domestic product (GDP) on health care than other countries and has 2.5 times the average health expenditure per capita than the Organization for Economic Cooperation and Development (OECD) and far exceeds the lower bound (Figure 6.1). In 2012, 18% or $3 trillion of the US GDP was spent on health-care services.

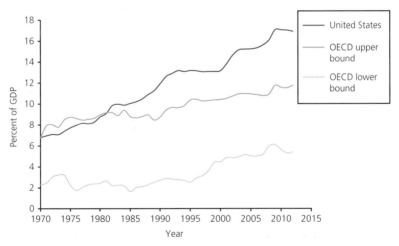

Figure 6.1 Health expenditure—percent of gross domestic product.

One reason for this disparity can be explained by the manner in which health-care services are paid in the United States. Prior to 1983, most health insurer, including Medicare and Medicaid, reimbursed providers under a fee-for-service system. Despite some limitations on how much and the frequency a provider could claim a service, the outcome rewarded volume and discouraged efficiency. The combination of fee-for-service, available health insurance, and the consumers' imperfect information about their health care created incentives for providers to provide and consumers to consume and a moral hazard that resulted in greater consumption health-care resources than would be the case in a competitive market.

ACA quality and outcome

Even though the United States spends more of its GDP on health care than other countries, the United States experiences unsatisfactory quality outcomes. The Institute of Medicine (IOM) *To Err is Human: Building a Safer Health System* highlights the issue of patient safety in US health care [4].The IOM reports that US citizens fare worse in areas such as diabetes, obesity, heart disease, chronic lung disease, infant mortality, and premature low birth weight babies [5]. Many of these conditions have a profound effect on young people that reduces the odds that Americans will live to age 50 and, for those who do, these conditions contribute to poorer health and greater illness later in life. The IOM reports on improving access and is charged to assess the current oral health-care delivery system; explore its strengths, limitations, and future challenges; and describe a vision for the delivery of oral health care to vulnerable and underserved population. The IOM reports that health-care quality and access are suboptimal especially for minority and low-income groups. For instance, in 2011, out of a population of 310 million, 59 million individuals were uninsured for at least part of the years, and 34 million individuals were uninsured for more than a year. The issue of equity and access to dental care is seen at the Mission of Mercy, a large-scale dental clinic that is held annually in many states, where hundreds queue for hours for a single weekend of free dental care.

The Agency for Healthcare Research and Quality (AHRQ) publishes annual reports on health-care quality, but they don't report on dental measures. Quality outcome measures in dentistry remain in the formative stages compared to medicine. Dental care quality measures are in the process of development but currently focus on process and treatment metrics rather than outcome measures. Each year since 2003, AHRQ has reported on the progress and opportunities to improve health-care quality and reduce health-care disparities. As mandated by the Congress, the National Healthcare Quality and Disparities Report focuses on national trends in the quality of health care provided to the American people. The report focuses on prevailing disparities in health-care delivery as it relates to racial factors and socioeconomic factors in priority populations.

ACA themes

A number of themes underlie health-care reform and the ACA. The prevailing theme is Donald Berwick's Triple Aim that frames an optimized health system. The Triple Aim looks to improve the health of the population, improve the experience of care for the patient, and reduce the cost of care. To improve health means better outcomes as measured by the absence of dental disease rather than high-tech treatment of the disease itself. To improve the experience of the patient is to put the patient in the center of care, not the dentist. And the quality of the process and the quality of the outcome are to be achieved at a lower cost of care than the current cost.

Crossing the Quality Chasm provides a starting strategy to improve the health system's quality of care: safe, effective, patient centered, timely, efficient, and equitable [6]. First, care is safe and avoids injury from the care that is intended to help. The service is effective and based on scientific knowledge to all who can benefit and refrains from services to those not likely to benefit—it is not all the personal preference of the dentist. The care is patient centered and respectful of and responsive to the patient's preference, need, and value, and ensures the patient's value guides clinical decisions. The care is timely and harmful delays are reduced. The care is efficient and avoids waste, including waste of equipment and supplies. And, lastly, the care is equitable and does not vary in quality. In short, the IOM's recommendation places the patient at the center of the dental care universe that was formerly occupied by the dentist.

The theme of value of health care is based on outcomes, not process: what happens and not what is done. The current system of health care rewards higher volume of treatment and higher cost services. The implant service is favored over the prevention service. The current system is a zero-sum competition where the incentives are not aligned to produce the best value for the consumer of health-care services. Value-based health care moves away from fee-for-service toward bundled payment and payment for outcome. The competitive value-based health-care system focuses on per dollar cost expended based on health conditions over the full cycle of care and health-care payments that align with health-care outcomes.

The overarching ACA theme is to integrate a fragmented health-care system to increase equity of access to care and promote positive health outcomes: dentists fulfilling their social covenant. The theme expands dental care to integrate oral health into general health to avoid waste in overlapped systems, share health information across silos, and utilize nondentist providers to screen for disease, assess risk, and provide anticipatory preventive care.

Actuarial value

Health plans in the individual and small group markets provide health coverage that meets certain distinct price levels. The levels of coverage are based on a percent of the actuarial value of the plan. The actuarial value is the expected percent of the plan's reimbursed medical expenses for the EHB for a standard population. These are commonly tiered into metal levels. The metal levels are platinum, gold, silver, and bronze with corresponding actuarial value of 90, 80, 70, and 60%. The actuarial values for a stand-alone dental plan are high and low with 85% and 70%, respectively.

Health plans purchased by individuals and small businesses on the health exchange will have similar plan designs with different price points. With no other information available, consumer purchases are influenced by brand and price. Price is king on the health-care marketplace. But consumers will have access to much more information to judge insurance products, providers, and provider networks as the quality metric provisions of the ACA kick into play.

ACA dental benefit

Pediatric dental benefit plans can be offered on a health-care exchange as an embedded plan, bundled plan, or a stand-alone plan. When the health insurer embeds the pediatric dental benefit, the health plan is presented as a single policy, and premium covers all 10 EHB. The embedded pediatric dental plan is integrated within the health plan and is not separately branded. When the health insurer bundles the pediatric dental benefit into its health plan, the health plan offers two distinct insurance policies sold together as a package. A bundled or embedded plan is easily submerged in the health plan and is not readily seen by the member. A stand-alone pediatric dental benefit plan is sold as a separate offering and is distinct from the health plan. A stand-alone plan requires the consumer to separately sign up for the stand-alone product and pay a separate premium. The stand-alone pediatric dental benefit puts another layer to acquire health benefits in an already complicated process. But a stand-alone plan offers more exposure to the consumer for dental care and dental-specific customer. Connecticut, Vermont, and the District of Columbia offer only embedded dental insurance plans. New York, Colorado, and Massachusetts offer a choice of insurance with or without embedded dental and a stand-alone option.

The ACA treats dental insurance for children and adults differently. Dental coverage for children is an essential health benefit that must be offered to the consumer but is not required to be purchased by the consumer. Dental insurance for adults is not mandatory. So, while health insurance is mandatory for everyone, dental insurance is not mandatory for anyone, even for children. This is a significant shortcoming of the ACA design.

Impact on dentistry

The ACA requires health plans to develop quality improvement strategies and implement quality assurance program to evaluate appropriateness and quality of covered services. Quality assessment in dental care is relatively undeveloped when compared to medicine, and the dental measures are little changed in the past three decades. A description of quality assessment measures in private dental practice shows no widely accepted standardized measures of treatment outcomes that leaves the dental profession not prepared to assess the quality of care in the current system and compare the quality of care in alternative models of dental care delivery. There are multiple reasons that contribute to the limited efforts to develop dental quality assessment methods and measures. Some interrelated reasons for the limited set of dental care assessment tools available can be traced to the historic development of the profession, the manner in which dentists are trained and licensed, reliance on procedure codes rather than a diagnosis codes, and the experience-based rather than an evidence-based view of dental treatment.

Some validated quality measures exist today. The Consumer Assessment of Healthcare Providers and Systems (CAHPS) is a consumer survey that measures the patient satisfaction experience with the dental office, dentist, and dental plan. CAHPS can measure consumer satisfaction on the dentist level up to the dental benefit company level. The Health Plan Employer Data and Information Set (HEDIS) includes one dental measure applicable to Medicaid members. Oral health quality of life measures exists today like the Early Childhood Oral Health Impact Scale, Geriatric Oral Health Assessment Index, Oral Health and Quality of Life Instrument, and Oral Health Impact Profile. When these measures are administered pretreatment and posttreatment, they provide an assessment of a treatments impact on a patient's quality of life.

In 2009, the Centers for Medicare and Medicaid Services proposed that the Dental Quality Alliance (DQA) develop performance measures for oral health. DQA's mission is to advance performance measurement to improve oral health with the objective to identify and develop evidence-based oral health measures and foster professional accountability and transparency. The DQA programmatic measure set 1 looks at utilization, quality of care, and cost for pediatric dental care (Table 6.2). The measures are process in nature to show the proportionate treatments delivered to a population (Table 6.3). The DQA quality measures are limited to those where the data can be derived from dental claims. The ultimate goal is to determine whether the recommended evidence-based treatment actually reduces dental disease over time.

Quality assessment like the DQA and CAHPS measured on the health plan and the provider level provides measures to be compared to benchmarks. Quality assessment can compare standardized, valid measures between different sets of providers (dentist, dental group, nondentist provider) and systems (dental plan, teledentistry, accountable care organization, dental–medical partnership).

These baby steps are essential to take as the dental profession moves to evidence and outcome-based quality measures. Dental delivery and payment systems will be built around quality assessment and quality assurance.

Table 6.2 Dental quality alliance programmatic measure set 1. (http://www.ada.org/~/media/ADA/Science%20and%20Research/Files/dqa-pediatric-measure-set-rfp.ashx)

Purpose	Measure	Domain
Utilization	Use of services	Use
Utilization	Preventive services	Use
Utilization	Treatment services	Use
Utilization	Emergency department	Outcome
Utilization	Emergency department—follow-up	Process
Quality of care	Evaluation	Process
Quality of care	Topical fluoride	Process
Quality of care	Sealant 6–9 years	Process
Quality of care	Sealant 10–14 years	Process
Quality of care	Continuity of care	Process
Quality of care	Usual source of care	Process
Cost	Per member per month	Cost

Reproduced with permission from the DQA. © 2012.

Table 6.3 Dental quality alliance measure set specifications (http://www.ada.org/~/media/ADA/Science%20and%20Research/Files/NQF_Dental_DQA_Topical_Fluoride.ashx)

	Fluoride	Sealant	Evaluation	Utilization
Age	≤21	6–9 10–14	≤21	≤21
Numerator	Two applications	First or second molar	Comprehensive or periodic	At least one service
Denominator	Enrolled	Enrolled	Enrolled	Enrolled
Aggregation	Health plan	Health plan	Health plan	Health plan
Domain	Process	Process	Process	Process
IOM aim	Equity Effective	Equity Effective	Equity Effective	Equity

Reproduced with permission from the American Dental Association. © 2015.

Cost of care

Consumers will increasingly rely on quality measures to select a dental plan, dental system, and dental provider. Consumer-driven competition will drive lower cost of care. One DQA measure in its starter set of metrics is the cost of care. The push from the ACA for accountable and transparent care at a lower cost of care will ripple through the dental care system. The impact of the ACA will foster new systems of dental care that may foster a movement away from the small dental practice, fee-for-service model toward integrated care, accountable care organizations, bundled payment, or pay for performance systems. Higher reimbursement levels may be offered to those who can show measurable high-quality, effective, appropriate, and cost-efficient dental care. The new, emerging dental delivery models promise to deliver on the promise of the Triple Aim.

ACA implication for dentists

The forecast for dentistry is that children are the growth segment to generate new patient flow into the practice. General dentists who are adept to treat children will thrive. Adult dental visits and dental income have remained flat for a decade, and general dentists that continue to compete for the shrinking segment struggle and begin to incorporate nondental cosmetic services like dermal fillers in an effort to be relevant. However, on the flip side, by 2018, it is forecast that the ACA will add 8.7 million new children with dental insurance coverage to the market with 3 million through Medicaid expansion, 3 million through the health insurance exchange, and 3 million through the employer-sponsored insurance for small employer plans [7]. The increased number of insured children promises to generate an additional $4 billion in dental spending [8].

Besides expanding the practice to treat children, dentists must move to lower their operating cost to remain competitive and grow. Unlike the anticipated fee increase for primary care physicians, dentists should not look to the ACA to increase fees. It is more likely that the maximum allowable fee for dental services will remain at the current state Medicaid fee level. Moreover, the fee-for-service payment model becomes irrelevant when the ACA's theme of quality performance disengages from fee-for-service and adopts alternative payment models. Dentists, dental groups, and dental systems that anticipate the change to patient demographic and the change in dental payment models will continue to thrive.

Change is inevitable and change is happening. Quantifiable quality of care and cost efficiency count, and the new dentist that demonstrates these attributes will be as busy as ever when employers and consumers armed with more information move toward health-care delivery models that promote these attributes [9]. The new generation of dentist pre-positions themselves into groups or systems that allows them to deliver dental care as part of a team in accountable care organization configurations that emphasize coordination in global payment models (Chapter 9).

Other than coordinated dental care, dental practices that deliver on the concept of medical–dental integration will become the dental home and the primary source of dental care in their community. The ACA supports integration of oral health care into general health care, where there is ample opportunity to share health contact opportunities between medicine and dentistry to the benefit of the consumer. For instance, the annual medical checkup may not have as much value as track and report blood pressure trends at multiple times at multiple venues like the dental appointment. The bidirectional nature of some systemic conditions, like diabetes, lends itself to a close medical–dental connection.

To have multiple points of contact in a coordinated health system that includes medical–dental integration is a benefit to the consumer.

Pediatric specialist extenders

The current dental workforce is ill prepared to address the increase of children who are newly eligible for dental care through the ACA and Medicaid expansion. The safety net system of federally qualified health centers and community health centers does not have the capacity to serve the children who are unable to access private practice dental care. If there is a lack of general dentists that treat children, there is also a lack of pediatric dentists who participate in the Medicaid program. Only 14 of 39 states have more than 50% of dentists treat Medicaid patients, and only 1 of 41 states has more than 50% of dentists that treat more than 100 patients on an annual basis. The dental profession fails its responsibility to care for the public's oral health.

The pediatric dentist specialist is trained to handle the highest need and the most complicated cases. But only 3% of the 200,000 professionally active dentists are pediatric dentists. General dentists receive as little as 2 weeks of formal training in dental school to treat children. It's no wonder that they are oftentimes uncomfortable to treat children, particularly very young children.

A new role for the pediatric dentist specialist is necessary because the current dental workforce is not up to the task to fill the need. In this scenario, the pediatric dentist takes on the role of a teacher, trainer, manager, and mentor to general dentists who treat children in a group practice, dental system, integrated accountable care organization, or community health center. The general dentist treats the majority of children who don't require the specialist care. The children will squirm but don't require the specialist's care. In addition to being the manager of pediatric care, the pediatric dentist specialist is then free to treat those children who absolutely require a specialist. The child is integrated into a system of anticipatory care under the aegis of a specialist and then is transferred to adolescent and adult care in the same facility. The current system of shifting a child between offices and providers is transformed into a coordinated pediatric dental care delivery system. The pediatric dental specialist now can extend their skill and expertise to a greater number of children.

Society's expectations

Dental care is seen as a public good, and society expects that the health professional will work in the interest of the public's health. Dentists have an obligation to care for the public's oral health and improve access to care. However, society is examining its relationship with the dental profession and finds it wanting; it doesn't feel fairly treated in the social covenant.

Society perceives an imbalance of the social contract in that practitioners of dentistry receive more than they give and there are a large number of children who have no access to a dental home. There is a view that the barrier to dental care access continues because the dental profession lacks advocacy for access to dental care for low-income individuals; dental organizations are poor advocates for access to dental services by Medicaid and CHIP beneficiaries: the organized dentistry is self-serving when they lobby for increased fees; the dental profession provides false leadership and lip service when it comes to issues about dental care for low-income individuals; some public policy makers from every state share negative feelings about dentists; and some state legislators believe that dentists have failed in their community service obligation to participate in Medicaid and CHIP [10, 11]. In a further blow to the self-esteem of dentists, a survey was conducted in Colorado to ascertain the most credible dental representative to deliver oral health messages. The community group was receptive to many messengers except the dentist because in this community, dentists are viewed as affluent and self-serving and not at all credible.

This is not to say that dentists and the profession are uncaring. In our experience, this is not so. But for many, perception is reality. It's incumbent upon dentists and the dental profession to maintain or regain the trust of the public and fulfill their social covenant. As the ACA and Medicaid expansion extends dental benefits to a wider base of consumers, dentists must position themselves to deliver on the promise of cost-effective, quality care in new delivery settings.

Interested readers are referred to Reference [12] as well.

Conclusion

The Patient Protection and ACA along with Medicaid expansion and CHIPRA is the most significant change in the financing and delivery of health care that this generation has experienced. The ACA is the driver for health-care reform that will reverberate through the dental profession, at least through the next generation of practitioners. More and more citizens will have access to dental benefits that may not be purchased from their employer. The payers of care will look to cost-efficient care with demonstrable quality and positive outcomes. The federal government through health-care exchanges and direct subsidies will drive the payer market. Dental care in the not too distant future will be delivered to the consumer in ways other than the small, private practice. Group practice, group systems, integrated care, coordinated care, and medical–dental integration are the manner in which dentists will practice in the future. This is the new normal.

The ACA enrollment targets are being met, and different constituencies are introducing innovative models of care that address the challenge. In the short term, dental care and dentistry are not affected in either the payment or care delivery system. But it's incumbent upon the generation of entering dentists to understand the new normal and adjust the working model of dental care. The ACA introduces a multitude of challenges and also a multitude of opportunity for every dentist.

The ACA sets the stage for a more inclusive health system that is accountable and transparent, measures quality, and strives to be cost efficient. The ACA supports innovation in the health-care workforce and in health-care delivery. Dentists who elect to stand by the wayside to continue business as usual as the health system evolves will soon find themselves marginalized and irrelevant. Those that embrace the new normal will find challenge, fulfillment, and success as the reward for improving the health of the communities that they serve.

References

1 Patient Protection and Affordable Care Act 2010. 2010 Public Law 111-148, 111th Congress 2010. http://www.gpo.gov/fdsys/pkg/PLAW-111publ148/pdf/PLAW-111publ148. pdf (accessed November 1, 2014).

2 The Patient Protection and Affordable Care Act Detailed Summary. Democratic Policy & Communications Center. http://www.dpc.senate.gov/healthreformbill/healthbill04.pdf (accessed November 1, 2014).

3 Health Care and Education Reconciliation Act of 2010. Public Law 111-152, 111th Congress 2010. http://www.gpo.gov/fdsys/pkg/PLAW-111publ152/pdf/PLAW-111publ152. pdf (accessed November 1, 2014).

4 Kohn LT, Corrigan JM, Donaldson MS. *To err is human: building a safer health system*. National Academy Press, Washington, DC, 1999.

5 US Health in International Perspective – Shorter Lives, Poorer Health. Institute of Medicine, 2013. http://www.iom.edu/~/media/Files/Report%20Files/2013/US-Health-International-Perspective/USHealth_Intl_PerspectiveRB.pdf (accessed November 1, 2014).

6 Committee on Quality of Health in America. *Crossing the quality chasm: a new health system for the 21st century*. National Academy Press, Washington, DC. 2001.

7 Nasseh K, Vujicic M, O'Dell A. Affordable Care Act Expands Dental Benefits for Children But Does Not Address Critical Access to Dental Care Issues. American Dental Association 2013. http://www.ada.org/~/media/ADA/Science%20and%20Research/Files/HPRCBrief_0413_3.ashx (accessed November 1, 2014).

8 Options for Covered California to Offer Pediatric Dental Coverage in 2015. Covered California 2013. http://www.healthexchange.ca.gov/BoardMeetings/Documents/November%2021,%202013/Pediatric%20Dental%20Report.pdf (accessed November 1, 2014).

9 Bader JD. Challenges in Quality Assessment of Dental Care. *Journal of the American Dental Association* 2009; 140: 1456–1464.

10 Nash D. Societal Expectations and the Profession's Responsibility to Reform – the Dental Workforce to Ensure Access to Care for Children. *California Dental Association Journal* 2011; 39: 504–510.

11 Slavkin H. The Failure of Dentistry's Social Contract with America and California's Search for Legislative Solutions? *Journal of Dental Education* 2003; 67: 1076–1077.

12 Halvorson GC. *Health care will not reform itself*. CRC Press, New York, 2009.

PART III
Competitive Strategies

CHAPTER 7

Ethics and ethical behavior

Gary Herman

School of Dentistry, University of California, Los Angeles, USA

Introduction

Ethics and ethical behavior are a significant issue in dentistry. The issues that rise to the top are the educational debt a dentist carries into their professional lives and how that debt may shade their treatment plan decision in a fee-for-service benefit system that rewards the quantity of services delivered. In a letter-to-the-editor segment, a recent prosthodontics resident opined that he feared that debt will shade treatment plan decisions toward higher revenue procedures [1]. A small-scale review of 100 high-revenue practices showed that over a 2-year period, the number of patients declined and the cost per patient rose (M. Okuji, pers comm, January 2015). Another issue that is emerging is that a significant portion of the US population that never before held dental benefits will gain new dental benefits through aspects of the Affordable Care Act. The ethics and ethical behavior issue that may surface is whether a two-tiered dental delivery system will arise where holders of different levels of dental benefits will receive different levels of care based on reimbursement levels.

Although this book is focused on looking into the future of the delivery of dental care, it is not possible to discuss ethics without spending a little time looking back. Dentistry in America has progressed from an itinerant trade to a cottage business to a modern health-care discipline with its ethical foundation more or less intact, but not without some conflicts. The good news is that the ethical principles are still relevant and vital enough to be useful to develop ethical positions in new circumstances.

What is a profession?

The dictionary simply defines a profession as a paid occupation, especially one that involves prolonged training and a formal qualification. Using that definition, dentistry certainly qualifies, but so do many occupations, including, perhaps,

Dental Benefits and Practice Management: A Guide for Successful Practices, First Edition.
Edited by Michael M. Okuji.
© 2016 John Wiley & Sons, Inc. Published 2016 by John Wiley & Sons, Inc.

beauticians and building contractors. In health care, professionalism not only includes mastery of a complex subject but also touches on the rights that accompany being a member of the profession and the responsibilities that are attached. As a result, most health professions have a form of self-governance and ethical codes.

In today's world, having my coffee brewed this morning from a professional barista, having arrived at the office courtesy of a professional cabbie, and looking at the social media coupon of a fellow dentist for a professional "examination, cleaning, and x-rays, regularly 300 dollars, only 29 dollars, new patients only," it is understandable that the definition of a profession is a bit flexible. What distinguishes dentistry is the commonly held belief that dentists have an obligation to use their knowledge and skills, first and foremost, to benefit their patients above providing for their own benefit.

As the economics of dentistry continue to change, additional pressure will be applied to members of the profession to focus on the commercial aspects of patient care. How dentists choose to respond to these changes will be instrumental to determine whether we are still worthy of calling ourselves professional.

A true profession demands that the nonprofessional we deal with, whether patients or others, be treated with respect and honesty.

Ethical versus legal

When I discuss ethics and ethical issues with dentists and dental students, it is common for a question to begin "Is it legal to...?" Ethics and the law are very different subjects, but it is surprising how often they are thought of as two aspects of the same subject. As well-known lawyer and business ethicist Michael Josephson says, "The law tell us what we can't do (prohibitions) and, sometimes what we must do (mandates); it does not answer the bigger question of what should we do?"

An ethical principle is inherently more basic than law. Because an ethical principle generally represents a cultural consensus, they are not judged against another standard. A law can be judged, generally, against an ethical standard. It is possible for a law to be unethical, but an ethical principle is neither legal nor illegal. Two problems exist for the practicing dentist: first, to become familiar with the laws that govern the practice of dentistry, and second, to make sure that the law makes ethical sense.

When an analysis of enforcement actions by state dental boards is undertaken, it is an easy exercise to see the correlation between the legal violation and an underlying specific ethical breach. Gross negligence and incompetence are clearly failing the principle of nonmaleficence—not doing harm. Fraudulent billing and misleading advertising fly in the face of the principle of veracity—truthfulness. It can be claimed that if dental practitioners performed all of their duties completely ethically, there would be no need for a Dental Practice Act. It is probably just as valid to reason that dental laws have been enacted primarily because some dentists have previously failed to act ethically.

The biggest difference that I see is the motivation for ethics and for laws. Ethical principles, codes of conduct, and advisory opinions are derived from individual and collective group decisions about what is the right thing to do. On the other hand, laws are enacted to require specific behaviors or prevent specific actions and to carry weight by threat of punishment. Ethical behavior is ultimately self-directed and done out of a sense of what is right. Laws are other-directed and followed out of a sense of duty or out of a concern for potential punishment.

While few dentists ever fully memorize the Dental Practice Act, just following Principles of Ethics accomplishes the same result.

Ethics and professionalism

Having defined profession and discussed ethics a bit, I believe it is important to devote a little time to the concept of professionalism. Professionalism includes ethical behavior but it is substantially more. The American College of Dentists, in its Ethics Handbook for Dentists, provides a charge to dentists to be professional. It stresses the need for dentists to place the patients' interests first and the need to respect the patients' values and preferences. Professionalism includes integrity, honesty, and competence. A professional has a responsibility to improve personally and to help the profession improve. A professional should support professional organizations and must be concerned about his/her own conduct as well as the perception of that conduct. Finally, a professional is ethical.

Ethics of quality of care

Within the practice of dentistry, the heart of professionalism lies in the delivery of high-quality dental care. Although this sounds rather simple, it is a complex issue made more so by the lack of absolute quality of care standards, the difficulty for patients to determine the quality of the care they received, and the vested interest of one practitioner to evaluate the work of another practitioner. In the legal arena of dentistry, to establish the standard of care is often critical when fleshing out a malpractice claim or determine a violation of the Dental Practice Act.

Ethically, the dentist has the responsibility to continue to monitor their own actions, procedures, and results to ensure that the dentistry provided is of quality that at least meets a commonly accepted standard. While a local dental society's peer review committee has manuals to help define good, acceptable, and bad dentistry, most dentists can easily examine a patient and make a value judgment about the quality of care delivered. If we can point out problems with previous dental care, we should be just as dedicated to make sure that our own dentistry, under self-assessment, meets those same standards.

In dentistry, there is a fairly broad range of treatment options that qualify as being within the standard of care. Problems occur when one dentist takes another dentist to task for practicing below the standard. That accusing dentist has a professional obligation to be truthful and provide the results of their examination. However, the accusing dentist has a competing obligation to not unnecessarily damage the reputation of a colleague.

It is important to remember that I believe the quality of care is a nebulous concept, influenced by the dentist's personal practice value, patient's expectation, changing technology, and social, economic, and cultural perspectives. That being said, if care is unnecessary, inappropriate, or clearly badly executed, it is below the quality standard.

It is difficult, but necessary, to balance the need to be truthful with patients and the desire not to denigrate another practitioner's treatment decision and outcome.

Perceptions of ethics and professionalism

Dentists are perceived, and judged, by their actions. Patients evaluate their dentist's skill by their total experience with the dentist and dental office. Patients don't usually think in terms of ethics. They evaluate their dentist based on the personal appearance of the dentist (Do they appear competent?) and the office appearance (Does it appear safe?) as well as the dentist's demeanor and confidence. Although it seems intuitive that a dentist is judged on their "gentleness," that is, whether there is pain or not, more likely the dentist is to be taken to task by their patient if it's not explained beforehand that it might be uncomfortable and if no empathy is displayed when something hurts.

In the health-care arena, "professional appearance" has been considered a significant factor in judging professionalism. In a dental school setting, although patients prefer a more formal attire for students and faculty to feel comfortable, other factors seemed to be as important. These factors included verbal skill, listening skill, and, interestingly, whether the student was wears too much perfume or cologne.

Although a patient cannot evaluate their dentist using the ethical principles of the profession, they can quickly and surely evaluate their dentist based on how they feel they are treated. To take the time to listen, explain, provide options, and establish a course of treatment that includes the best options for the patient ensures the greatest likelihood that the patient remains confident in their level of care.

Perception of ethical behavior by another professional is a different issue. Unlike a patient, a peer is likely to judge another peer based on the ethical principles. However, they may not express their opinion any more lucidly than a patient. A dentist is perceived as professional if they provide good quality care and communicate well with colleagues, especially if they collaborate on or refer mutual patients. A poor clinical outcome does not confer a poor professional reputation, but several poor outcomes without adequate interaction with the referring colleague likely will damage a reputation.

Situational ethics

The term situational ethics conveys the idea that ethical behavior is not absolute. Ethical behavior may be different under different conditions or circumstances. Hardcore ethicists often call this contextualism and philosophically argue that the concept of universal ethics is not particularly valid. Unfortunately, situational ethics has the potential to be misused to rationalize unethical behavior that is something akin to "the devil made me do it."

Responsibility to the patient

Ethically and legally, responsibility to your patients is the primary guiding principle for health-care professionals. We are trusted to have the knowledge, skill, and judgment to treat patients. We are entrusted with the duty to use those skills, first and foremost, to better the lives of our patients. This duty is a fiduciary duty. Some think a fiduciary duty is to make fiscally sound decisions and not steal or defraud others. That certainly is true, but further, a fiduciary duty is a requirement that our actions and decisions are in the best interest of the person or entity we have the fiduciary duty to, rather than ourselves or anyone or anything else.

In practice, it is convenient to think in terms of our relationship with a patient as a business contract. We do, in fact, have a contractual relationship. The patient is offered a set of services and a treatment plan with a hoped for, but not guaranteed, prognosis. In the fee-for-service system, the patient agrees to pay a specific sum for those services. That is the essence of a legal contract.

But we are not selling, nor are the patients buying furniture. A patient cannot meaningfully "shop" to evaluate the quality of a crown margin. Patients can only judge the dentist after the fact. Even then, their judgment is limited to rather subjective assessments. For this reason, dentists must, within the context of one's values, make a treatment plan choice and a treatment decision that is appropriate for the patient and provide that patient with the information to choose appropriately. That is the essence of an informed consent.

The wheels fall off when the dentist, consciously or otherwise, makes a treatment decision that discounts patient autonomy and limit choice for the patient in an effort to accomplish a marketing objective or to meet a production goal. This is when the dentist becomes a furniture salesman. Situational ethics is not rationalization to dispense with ethical principle when treating a patient.

Responsibility to improve health

I sit on a dental school admissions committee. Almost every admission application I have ever read includes either a neat list of humanitarian volunteer projects the applicant has been involved with or, at the least, a strong statement regarding the applicant's desire to help their fellow men by addressing health-care inequities once a degree and a license are obtained. I have become jaded over the years but still fully believe that most of our students enter health care as an opportunity to serve rather than just another job opportunity. There is a near universal desire to help patients achieve better health. Upon graduation, this notion seems to get a bit diverted by the desire to be gainfully employed and the need to repay staggering student debt. That level of indebtedness can certainly be considered a situation necessitating a modification of one's ethical beliefs, if it means a job. But is it right?

Marketing strategies abound in dentistry. A different practice philosophy is reasonable. There are ethical concerns when marketing strategies are designed to drive patients to a practice for a specific procedure, say, an implant or cosmetic veneer or Invisalign orthodontic appliance. Consumers are accustomed to comparison shop and may come to a dentist just for that specific procedure. If they do not wish to have a comprehensive workup and consider your desire to take appropriate radiographs and perform an examination as just a way of jacking up your price, are you willing to send the patient away, even though the advertising mailer costs a goodly amount of money to produce and mail?

But in this case of marketing a service, is it a case of bait-and-switch if one service is promoted and then an additional second service is required to receive the first service? Can a consumer be faulted for becoming skeptical of the additional service and fee even if they are legitimate and required? And finally, why are dentists surprised when the consumer reacts negatively to their professional advice and lower their esteem of the dental profession when they are lured by the promise of a service only to be told that high ethics and quality of care requires them to pay more than was plainly advertised?

If you, as a professional, wish to improve a patient's health, you must see a patient. If you cannot get patients into your waiting room, you cannot make the difference you wish to make. If getting patients into your office relies on a marketing approach that focuses on a specific procedure, you may make money, but you might not make a difference in the patient's health. You just complete a service.

As a dentist, you are responsible for the entire oral cavity and a bit more. You need to honor that responsibility.

Responsibility to family

We are, of course, talking about your family. Many of you have or will have families to provide for, deal with, and take into account along with your dental practice. I am reminded of a former student, then a new specialist, who asked my opinion about where he should look to locate. After a short conversation, I gathered that he was planning to buy a house, start a family, and buy or open a new practice, more or less simultaneously. After recommending professional counseling, I realized that he was giving himself a great motivational tool to succeed. He couldn't afford to fail. But how does that play out when professional ethics butts up against next month's mortgage payment?

Dentist as expert

One of the principal reasons why health care demands professional standards is the inherent conflict that arises from the fact that the dentist and the patient rarely share the same level of expertise about health care. Although I seem to have many patients who believe they know more about dentistry than I do, the reality is that patients must, at some level, trust the dentist to provide the information that the patient uses to make choices. If that information is inaccurate, inadequate, or just plain wrong, the patient cannot make good decisions. A dentist must have the objective qualifications like education, training, and knowledge and should have some intangible qualifications like confidence, assurance, and maybe a bit of charisma in order to be trusted readily by patients.

You're the doctor!

Over many years, I have come to dread the expression "You're the doctor" coming from a patient. It usually occurs after I have spent a considerable amount of time discussing my clinical finding with the patient and then presenting several well-thought-out treatment options including the risk, benefit, cost, and time needed for each option as well as discussing what could happen if no treatment is rendered. To hear a patient proclaim that I am the doctor is like getting a cream pie in the face. I already know that I am the doctor, and what the patient is really saying is "I don't really want to listen to all your hard work, just tell me what I should do." When this happens often enough, it becomes easier to shortcut the process, figuring the patient is likely to accept your preferred treatment option, because, as we all know, you're the doctor.

This is all the more reason for you *not* to succumb to this easy way out. The ethical principle of patient autonomy demands that the patient be given all of the information necessary to make a free and fully informed decision. The operative words are free and fully informed. "Free" refers to the lack of coercion or directing the presentation in a manner to accomplish a specific outcome. "Fully informed" means to provide all of the choices with all of the risks, benefits, and costs of the alternatives. Failing to provide all appropriate options or strongly skewing the presentation to achieve your desired choice subverts the patient's basic right. In a time when dentists are under greater financial pressures due to external forces seemingly out of their control, acting to direct the treatment plan process to the conclusion that is in the dentist's financial best interest rather than the patient's best interest is a serious slippery slope that can lead to unfortunate outcomes for both the dentist and their patient.

Take the high road and provide your patients with the information to make good decisions for themselves.

Dentist as estimator and advisor

As your patient's principal expert in oral conditions and care, your primary role as diagnostician is paramount. Your patient expects to be told what is wrong with their oral health. Additionally, they expect to be given information on how their problems can be corrected. It would be nice if dentists just stop there. We would not have to deal with pesky financial issues. It would be even better the tiring work of delivering dental treatment is delegated to someone else. Alas, that generally won't be happening anytime soon.

Many practice management experts suggest that you should be the advisor and diagnostician, but you should stay "above" the demeaning aspect of discussing fees and finances with patients. They recommend that you have a treatment coordinator, the closer, who discusses fees for treatment and makes financial arrangements. Others, including myself, believe it is appropriate for the dentist to acknowledge the fees and that dentistry has a cost and, therefore, a value. If you can comfortably mention the cost of treatment, without apology, it is easier for a patient to accept your fees as reasonable. If a patient believes that you do not know or care about the cost of treatment, it could be hard for them to accept that you care about them. That being said, it is probably better if you do delegate specific financial arrangements and discussions about dental benefit coverage to a staff member. Whichever way you choose to handle the financial arrangement, make sure you actually handle them. One of the biggest areas of conflicts between the patient and the dentist is miscommunication or failure to discuss costs of treatment.

Self-interest

Dental ethicists often talk about preferred patterns of practice. These patterns are the sum of an individual dentist's training, both in school and afterward, and the results of that dentist's clinical experience tempered by patient feedback. It is an important factor in determining treatment plans for patients; however, it should not be the overriding factor. Of higher importance is the health, both general and oral, of the patient and the patient's ability to be the dental decision maker. What you *want* to do is nice to know, but what the patient chooses to do, given enough information, is much more important. Currently, many practitioners respond to changes in the dental marketplace by making treatment recommendation choices that are clearly more about what is better for their pocket book than a patient's well-being.

The effect of establishing a pattern of practice that is unethical, by limiting patient knowledge, misrepresenting facts, or omitting options to either increase the revenue from expensive treatment or work around a dental benefit limitation, results in short-term benefit for a practitioner and causes serious problems in terms of professional liability and dental board action, as well as a broader concern with the level of trust in the dental profession by the public. It is essential that a patient be given choices and the power to decide on treatment.

Pattern of practice

Although we talked about practice patterns in the last section, we will look at this issue in a bit more detail. Let's start with the idea that there is, at a given time, only one standard of care. The concept of a standard of care is a bit like pornography: you have trouble defining it, but you know it when you see it. A standard of care may be fluid, certainly different now than 10 or 20 years ago, and it usually rests on generalities about what the average or prudent individual would do in the same situation. That being said, it is often quite easy to look at an action or a treatment choice or an outcome and say that it is within the standard of care or not. The biggest issue is whether the standard of care applies to all in your practice equally. Would you have some trouble making a case that you are practicing at the standard if you treat different segments of your practice differently if, for example, new patients with dental benefits routinely receive a full-mouth set of radiographs at the time of initial diagnosis, but noninsured patients only receive bitewing radiographs and two anterior periapical radiographs? What is your standard of care? Or are full crowns recommended to insured patients and three surface fillings for those with the same clinical presentation but no insurance? Is one group overtreated or the other group undertreated? What is your standard of care?

If patients respond to your flyer for a discounted new patient "deal," should they receive a different service than your full cash paying patients or your patients with dental benefits? Patients deserve to be treated equally, or they are not being treated fairly.

Ethical practice decisions

In ethics lectures and discussions, I often suggest that every decision about the practice is an ethical decision. Who you hire, what hours the office is open, and even the laboratory service you engage have, as a result, an effect on the patients' well-being and autonomy.

Because ethics are, at their best, aspirational, they differ from legal requirements that are quite prescriptive. Ethical decisions about practice operations cannot necessarily be the primary factor on how a practice is run, but rather should be a safety check. I recommend that a practice owner should periodically review their operations to make sure that a business decision, made principally to maintain practice's viability and increase profitability, has not created an ethical breach or conflict.

All too often I hear stories of practices that began with great intentions and a strong ethical footing that, over time, react to economic stresses by altering the practice model. Advertising, including "lost leader" specials and "free" services, lowering fees to increase volume, and hiring less qualified staff, as well as changes in treatment planning options can all have an impact on the ethics of the practice.

Most dentists who have developed serious ethical issues that have developed into Dental Practice Act problems did not begin their practices with the intent to be unethical. They usually relate that they altered the practice to remain in business or, occasionally, to make what they considered a reasonable amount of money for the time spent. This was a change to the business model that caused a change in the ethics. It is truly uncommon to hear a dentist say that he changed his ethical model and the business practices changed as a result. Business is business, but in dentistry, ethics is a part of doing business, not an afterthought.

The importance of profitability

There is no doubt that profitability is a goal of each and every private practice ever begun. If the overarching goal of the practice is to provide dental care to a population, an unprofitable practice cannot achieve that goal. The biggest concern occurs when making money becomes the only goal of the practice. Making money in the service of patients is markedly different than making money at the expense of patients.

Practice management seminars can focus on efficiencies of practice, patient acquisition, or treatment presentation skills. The underlying message is that managing the practice better will result in more patients served and more profitability. The pitfall for dentists is that by concentrating on managing the practice, patient service gets kicked to the curb by failing to provide accurate information or provide no information for a patient to make an informed decision or, at its worst, provide misinformation to accomplish the goal of profitability. To have a profitable dental business is necessary, but not at the cost of ethics.

Owner versus employee

It does not take a rocket scientist to figure out that the action, responsibility, and motivation of an employee dentist differ markedly from those of an owner dentist. Any dentist who has worn both of hats would undoubtedly agree. This section touches on the ethical challenges faced by the employee dentist in the employee–employer relationship.

Employee in a small private practice

For lack of a better word, I refer to the long-standing practice model of a solo or partner ownership of a practice in a relatively small office with few staff members. When this type of practice decides to expand, the thought is to hire a younger, less experienced practitioner to meet the increased patient flow of the practice. The associate typically takes over routine procedures to free up the experienced practitioners to provide specialized and more lucrative procedures. Sometimes, the associate is being auditioned for future ownership in the practice.

It should be remembered by all of the parties that this employment relationship requires a lot of effort to keep it intact. Inherent differences in status, relationship with the staff, and individual expectations make clear communication of paramount importance if problems are to be prevented or solved.

The ethical challenge for the associate occurs if the owner dentist has allowed unethical practices to develop in the office. An ethically conflicted associate is an unhappy associate. The choices for the associate are to accept and participate in the ethical breach, try to discuss the problem with the employer and effect a change (good luck with this approach), or quit and find a new job. It should be obvious that each of these options will create a boatload of stress for the employee dentist. The employee dentist in this type of relationship must focus on strong, open communication to prevent the escalation of the internal problem to an external legal issue.

Employee in large group practice

Associate dentists hired into a large group have all of the same potential issues found in the traditional practice. The difference is that the problems are likely to be magnified in the large group. Multidoctor offices are characterized by having much larger staff and additional layers of management that are nondentists. The principal owners tend to focus on the delivery of care, delegating running the practice to a business manager or a very powerful office manager.

In a small practice, the associate only has to convince the owner dentist and a couple of assistants that he knows something. In a large group, there is an entire battalion that has to be convinced. Many times, the nondentist management makes business decisions without understanding the legal or ethical requirements of the profession. It can be very difficult for the associate to get past that layer to inform the owner dentists of a problem. A dentist in a large group practice is well served to appear nonthreatening to the staff and management when confronted with situations that cause them concern.

Employee in a public health setting

An increasingly popular option for newer dentists is to work in a public health dental facility. These can include Federally Qualified Health Centers (FQHC), private charitable clinics, and government-run operations like the Indian Health Service and the Bureau of Prisons. Based on the purpose to serve an otherwise underserved population, this model seems less affected by ethical challenges. There are, however, still some potential issues.

Funding and payment structures tend to differ markedly from the private practice model. Often, revenue is based on a projected and expected level of service rather than the usual fee-for-service model. An FQHC may be reimbursed on a flat fee for each visit regardless of services provided. A prison is likely given a fixed annual budget. A charitable clinic may rely on foundation grants and donations from year to year.

Dentist may be paid an annual fixed salary regardless of productivity. Oversight and accountability can vary in these operations. This structure may make it easy to deliver less than optimum care or less than significant quantity of care to these deserving populations. There are definitely ethical considerations at play in this scenario. A dentist must remember that this is more than a job.

Employee in a dental support organization

Whether you call it a dental support organization (DSO), corporate practice, or something else, this model for dental care delivery is a fast-growing sector. This model has potential for ethical angst among the employee dentists. I would certainly not wish to suggest that all DSOs are unethical any more than I could state that all private practitioners place ethical practices at the top of their to-do lists. It has been documented that a number of these offices use questionable advertising, participate in upselling, and fail to provide the information needed by the patients to make a free and fully informed decision. An employee dentist, or even an owner dentist, will have many of the same issues as in the group practice with regard to administration and oversight, coupled with the likelihood that production demands may stress the dentist to consider unethical actions. It is probable that the idea to question the corporation policy is tantamount to tendering a resignation.

Recently, the formation of an association of these DSOs has resulted in the development of a code of ethics for these corporate entities related to the business management side of the practice. The question is why should there be a separate code of ethics for dentist in different practice settings.

Dental board

It is appropriate that in a discussion of ethics and ethical behavior, state dental boards that oversee dentists should be included in the discussion. Technically, there are no ethical issues before the state dental board. They exist to protect the public by licensing dentist and dental auxiliaries. Additionally, they enforce the laws related to the practice of dentistry. The rationale to include state dental boards is that while ethical is not the same as legal, the basis is the same. Nearly every single ethical code violation is also codified as a violation of a Dental Practice Act. Unethical actions are probably also illegal under state statute and can ultimately lead to censure, suspension, or revocation of a dental license.

As someone who personally knows members of my state's dental board as well as the investigators and prosecutors who work for the dental board, I can make two unequivocal statements: First, these individuals are very nice, personable individuals. Second, I never want to be the object of their attention in their official capacity. The dental board takes their mandate to protect the public by enforcing the Dental Practice Act very seriously. When the investigators discover a case with merit, they will pursue the case tenacious seriousness of purpose.

Many dental boards are self-funded, meaning that their operating revenue comes from only the funds derived from licensing fees, examination fees, and the recovery of the expenses for investigation from payments that arise from judgments and settlements of enforcement cases. They don't pursue frivolous claims.

Value of treatment alternatives

The ethical standard of informed consent and legal statues, confirmed by court rulings, specifically address the issue of treatment alternatives. If you have been in a hospital for a procedure, you have undoubtedly been asked to read and sign a long, detailed document that describes the procedure, alternative treatment, and potential risk, all of which must be acknowledged before any treatment begins. Although this disclosure is slower to develop dentistry, more dentists incorporate the written informed consent form into their practice. However, even with the written consent, there sometimes feels missing.

First, informed consent does not need to be a written document to be obtained. It is, however, always better to have a written and signed document. Second, to have a written and signed document is not a guarantee that informed consent is given.

The basic requirement for consent of a treatment plan includes a discussion of the examination findings and recommendations for treatment, including alternative treatment choice, risks and benefits of each course of treatment, cost of treatment alternatives, time needed to complete the alternative course of treatment, and, finally but very importantly, likely outcomes if no treatment is rendered. This is all quite difficult to deliver on a written form. The dentist may have a preferred treatment recommendation, but the patient deserves to have all appropriate options presented to them.

Standard of care

The term standard of care has been thrown around the dental profession for years both in dental education and dental litigation. There are differences in the term, standard of care, as it is applied into these two different realms. Among dentists, this concept is considered to be what their colleagues around them are doing. If their behavior is similar, they believe that they practice within the standard of care. Our legal colleagues have a bit less flexible standard. They refer to the establishment of a duty to care that is assumed when treating a patient. Failure to provide patients with care that is appropriate based on evidence and scientific research, current adopted practices, or otherwise justifiable places the dentist at risk for practicing below the standard.

Regardless of whose definition you choose, there is a reasonable series of actions and options based on your specific findings. While the definition of dental caries can result in several appropriate restorative options, most, if not all, dentists would consider prophylactic endodontic treatment and crown restoration for all cases of dental caries to be outside of the standard of care. My advice is to not overthink the standard of care, and if the treatment is reasonable, appropriate, and of adequate quality, then the treatment is within the standard of care.

Appropriate pattern of practice

The specific treatment recommended by the dentist is certainly influenced by that dentist's particular skill set, knowledge, experience, previous patients' acceptance, and overall success, based primarily on the very specific circumstances that lead to that individual dentist's view of the dental universe. I am aware of many of the newer technical advances of dentistry. I have chosen to adopt some techniques and technology and ignore, for the time being, others. The menu of techniques and technology that I offer to my patients is not set in stone. As I gain understanding, experience, and success, I will and have added new items to the menu. Just as all restaurants do not offer the same food items, not all dentists can or should offer all of the same treatment options.

Care must be taken to assure that the dentist's practice pattern does not infringe on the patient's rights to a fully informed consent. If I do not perform molar root canals, not giving the patient the option of the endodontic procedure, but rather only offering extraction and implant would certainly qualify as a violation of informed consent. As an example, recent restorative decisions related to metal-free restoration for all teeth speak to the evolution of standards of care and practice pattern that creates stress to the dental delivery system. Is a nonmetal restoration as effective and efficacious as a silver amalgam restoration and is there evidence that silver amalgam is detrimental to systemic health?

The wallet biopsy

There is an all-too-common business practice that can develop in a dental office, regardless of the business model. That is to perform the wallet biopsy to determine how much the traffic will bear when it comes to fees attached to a service. Whether it is cynically intentional or it happens out of laziness or the "I know best" attitude of the practitioners, failure to provide a thorough discussion of alternatives can lead to the perception that the diagnosis is based on financial consideration of the dentist rather than the patient's best interest. If one-treatment-fits-all approach is coupled with aggressive advertising, it can readily morph into the classic bait-and-switch type of marketing currently visible in an e-mail offer or on a billboard near you.

At its best, this approach to treatment planning is unethical. The failure to provide a free and fully informed consent is obvious. The patient is not being allowed to make a decision. Instead, the dentist has usurped that privilege. At its worst, this action is a callous business model designed to help a business to be successful. The patient is a consumer exploited to purchase the service that makes the most money for the business. In health care, if the marketing is untruthful, it violates legal statutes. The patient's best interest, not the provider's, is always the paramount ethical concern.

Social media and ethical behavior

Okay, I admit that the Internet is no longer a passing fad. There is little doubt that social media will become a larger influence in health care as the people who do not remember typewriters and correction fluids replace those of us who do remember these wonderful devices. The growing pain to adapt to new Internet social media sources is taking its toll on dental practice. In previous generations, an unhappy and aggrieved patient might tell a few of her friends and it stops there. The unhappy and aggrieved patient today is free to rant, rightly or wrongly, to thousands of readers over any number of social media websites designed for just such public disclosure. Social media creates the opportunity for a dentist to market their service, brand their persona, and get a message quickly and cheaply to many people. Social media also carries the risk of equally quick damaged reputation.

Social media is neither inherently ethical nor unethical. Social media does not change the definition of ethical behavior. Social media is both an advertising medium and a scorecard.

Will Yelp destroy a practice?

The answer to this question is yes, no, maybe, or all of the above. There is no question that social media has replaced most traditional advertising. The telephone book delivered to your door is dead as well as the yellow page business directory in the back. The issue is when a consumer looks for a dentist through a search engine and finds telephone numbers in their zip code, what do they really see? They may click on one of a dozen rating sites that give a star rating and comments from a number of reviewers. Is a two-star out of five-star rating based on one review from that patient whose new filling failed a week after being placed? Is the colleague's five-start rating based on five reviews sent in by their office staff? The lack of accountability and reliability of this information creates a problem for the dentist and patient alike. But this is what dentists are left with if they don't create an accountable and transparent rating alternative that includes patient satisfaction, dental care outcome, and cost of care criteria. For a dentist to say that these variables are solely in the ken of the professional and can't be quantified will leave social media as the arbiter of dentist quality of care.

Reputation repair is a new industry that social media has spawned where damaging reviews are removed and positive review inserted in order to raise a dentist's social media scorecard. The ethical concern arises when the repair involves falsehood, fabrication, and misstatement. To even respond to a negative comment must be done carefully, if at all, as it may violate a patient's privacy and may be considered a violation of HIPAA statute on patient privacy.

Dissemination of fees

The level of dental fees discussions has always been a touchy subject among dentists. Dentists are always concerned about their fees. Are they too high and possibly scaring away patients? Are they too low and give the perception of low quality? Are they the same as everyone else that makes it appear like merely mirroring their colleagues? Do dentists want to be perceived as a Nordstrom or a Target?

The ethical viewpoint might be whether the actual cost of care is considered when a fee is set or whether a fee is established based on the image a dentist wishes to convey. Is the practice to rob from Peter to give to Paul as when different fees are derived based on need or lack of need an ethical good? Are publically posted fees inherently consumer friendly or surfeit with possibility of self-diagnosis? Should a consumer be allowed to compare fees between dentists?

Most dentists have a fee but are comfortable to change that fee depending on the individual circumstance of the patient and the dentist. If I have a patient who requires additional time and energy due to their emotional make-up, I have no qualm to raise the fee. On the other hand, I willingly lower my fee if the patient's circumstances compel me to be benevolent. If my fees are widely public, I have difficulty explaining the difference of a higher but never the difficulty to explain the lower fee.

My opinion is that the public dissemination of fees brings more confusion to the consumer than clarity. The solution is simple. Clearly, thoroughly and truthfully discuss your fees with your patient as part of the treatment presentation. None of the other issues should matter at that point.

Future of dental ethics

I don't have a crystal ball. I have no special ability to see the future. I do know that a common way to attempt to assess the future is to look from the past to present and keep going. Change is inevitable. On the 150th anniversary of the American Dental Association's Principles of Ethics and Code of Professional Conduct, it is fitting to look at that document and realize how little the principles have changed since its inception. While changes to the Code of Professional Conduct have been well thought out and advisory opinions have been added and deleted to address changes in dental practice, the underlying document remains virtually intact. The principles of patient autonomy, doing well, not doing bad, being fair, and being truthful, remain a constant. New challenges to the ethical principles will undoubtedly continue to arise as technologies advance, new dental delivery models emerge, and the financing of dental care changes. New ethical challenges arise, but the ethical basis for resolution of these issues remains the same.

What is future ethical behavior?

If my premise is accurate, there are two answers to this question that have a decent shot of being correct. If the American Dental Association's Code of Professional Conduct and the Principles Ethics remain intact, there is a standard available by which to judge ethical behavior. The first answer is that ethical behavior is to put the patient first. The second answer to this question is ethical behavior will change due technical, scientific, and market forces in play. If self-regulation of the profession is weakened or replaced by governmental regulation related to health-care financing or governmental mandate, I suspect a very different picture of ethics could emerge. I believe in self-regulation by the profession that is embodied by the American Dental Association.

What is quality and who determines?

Quality is currently determined by the provider and the patient, as well as dental peers, insurance consultants, and occasionally paid dental expert witnesses. Quality in dentistry is like art. To define quality in dentistry has always been difficult. It can be patient satisfaction, but what do patients really know about what is in their mouth? It can be statistical information regarding health outcome. It can be assessment by a third party. Quality assessment will likely move away from patient satisfaction indices, which are hard to quantify, and probably move toward outcomes assessment. Financing by the government may hasten this move, as the Affordable Care Act will set parameters of outcomes and expected results as a reasonable way to define quality. This process seems potentially difficult to define, develop, and measure outcomes successfully. That's my crystal ball.

Conclusion

There is not one right answer.

If what you were looking for in this chapter was a specific directive on exactly what to do, ethically, I am truly sorry, as I know you are disappointed. My hope was for you to come away with a toolkit. These tools can help you ask the right questions, help you identify potential problems, and hopefully slow down your thought processes to allow for a thorough review of the important issues when making practice decisions. Remember that all practice decisions are ethical decisions.

Put the patient first is always the right decision.

Over the years, dentistry has tried to distill the ethical principles by describing them as the Golden Rule, or Commandments. I have heard the principles likened to the constitution, that is, a framework that allows for new interpretations without changing the underlying premises. I personally believe that what makes a health-care profession special is the responsibility to put the patient first in all of our decision making. Within that context, dentistry is one of the few professions, maybe the only profession that has included truthfulness as a specific ethical principle. Honoring the truth will allow you to ensure that the patient is an integral part of all your decision-making process.

Keep an open mind and a watchful eye.

When I reflect on my own journey through the profession, I realize that many of my decisions were made without a lot of deliberation. Some decisions happened despite me rather than because of me. Chance may have decided on a very different outcome.

I recommend that, with the many issues potentially affecting your careers, you try to make more educated decisions than I did. I understand that doing as I say rather than as I do is always difficult. Hopefully, the material presented in this chapter will help make the process easier. Above all, remember that dentistry is a wonderful profession and it is now your responsibility to keep it that way.

Reference

1 Letters: Student Loan Woes. *ADA News*. April 20, 2015; 46(8).

CHAPTER 8

Stay out of trouble

Matthew Cassady

Delta Dental of Colorado, Denver, USA

Introduction

By now, anyone reading this book likely has a decent grasp on what it means to be a dentist. You've toiled long and hard through years and years (and years and years) of school. You've passed your boards. Whether you're hanging your own shingle, going to work for the big shiny corporate practice with dozens of dentists, or planning to end up anywhere in between, you are ready to practice dentistry. You are ready to become the dentist you've always dreamed of being. Fill cavities, extract painful teeth, treat chronic periodontal disease—you name it, you can do it.

What most new dentists never envision, however, is the financial pressure that can come with choosing to become a dentist. In stark contrast to the idealist vision many have when they set out to become a dentist, the real world presents challenges unforeseen to most. Where once you only thought to treat patients, meet their needs, and leave them with a beautiful smile as evidence of their gratitude and your job well done, the real world demands that someone deliver the rent check, pay the receptionist, buy the dental chair, outfit the operatory, pay the hygienist, cover the lab bills, and still keep the lights on when everyone comes in tomorrow. Guess what, if you've hung your shingle and started your own practice, that person is you!

Even if you've gone to work for someone else, though, pressures other than those that come from treating patients are never far away. If the owner or manager of your practice is feeling the financial strain of running the practice, you will likely begin to feel that strain very soon as well. Several other pressures exist for employed dentists that have nothing to do with ensuring that patients receive proper care. Natural rivalries may exist that drive an upstart to outperform his fellow associate dentists. Obligations to a spouse, kids, or other family members mean that you can really use the extra money that would come from hitting a performance bonus. Then, there are the proverbial Joneses down the street who always seem to have the latest and greatest toys. How can you keep up?

Dental Benefits and Practice Management: A Guide for Successful Practices, First Edition.
Edited by Michael M. Okuji.
© 2016 John Wiley & Sons, Inc. Published 2016 by John Wiley & Sons, Inc.

The point is that no matter who you are and no matter where you practice, you almost certainly face pressures that drive you to increase production. These real or perceived benchmarks can create perverse incentives that drive even the most talented dentists to turn to creative avenues to meet them. In fact, an entire industry of practice managers and dental consultants has sprung up to aid dental practices to maximize their profits.

While many of these creative avenues to increase profitability constitute innovative methods by which to effectuate a viable, sustainable business in a changing economic climate, other creative avenues do not. This chapter addresses this latter category. The methods identified in this chapter fall into the categories of fraud, waste, or abuse. Any of these behaviors can land you into serious trouble. We want to help you stay out of trouble by identifying improper conduct and avoid it. We will tell you about the ill effects that fraudulent, wasteful, or abusive behavior can have and how it can adversely affect everyone involved, including you. Finally, we will discuss safeguards you can implement in your practice to ensure that fraud, waste, and abuse do not compromise your practice, your finances, or even your freedom.

Fraud, waste, and abuse

So what do we mean when we talk about fraud, waste, and abuse? If there are viable methods for increasing productivity and profit, how are they different from fraud, waste, and abuse? And how do you make sure you stay on the right side of that distinction? To answer these questions, we first need to define the terms. We will take each term in turn.

Fraud

Many different definitions exist for the term fraud. In general, fraud is deceit or trickery. Merriam-Webster's dictionary defines the term to mean the "intentional perversion of truth in order to induce another to part with something of value or surrender a legal right" or "an act of deceiving or misrepresenting" [1].

In a health-care setting, fraud has a considerably more specific meaning. The criminal provisions of the US Code have a very specific definition of health-care fraud: one that also comes with a penalty of up to 20 years in prison—even life in prison if the fraud results in the death of the victim (18 USC § 1347).

Medicaid's rules have a slightly different, though consistent, definition of fraud. The applicable section of the Code of Federal Regulations, 42 CFR § 455.2, states in pertinent part that fraud is "an intentional deception or misrepresentation made by a person with the knowledge that the deception could result in some unauthorized benefit to himself or some other person...."

Whatever specific definition one turns to for fraud, several things remain consistent. First, the person who commits fraud must deceive the victim of the fraud.

Second, the person who commits fraud must do so intentionally. If a person does not intend to deceive or trick the other person or entity, they have not committed fraud. What they have done may still be a crime or result in civil liability, but it cannot be fraud without intent. Finally, the actions of the person who commits the deception must result in a gain to the person doing the deceiving, a loss to the person being deceived, or both.

According to the *Economist*, fraud accounts for roughly 10% of Medicare and Medicaid spending and up to $272 billion nationwide [2]. Providers do not commit all of that fraud. Office staff, patients, insurance brokers, agents, and employer groups have all committed health-care fraud. Still, providers have the greatest opportunity to commit and remain accountable for most of the health-care fraud nationwide.

Waste

Of the three terms, fraud, waste, and abuse, the one that stumps most people is waste. What is it? Unlike fraud and abuse, no federal rule or regulation defines it. However, the National Association of Medicaid Directors points out that waste is "generally understood to encompass over utilization or inappropriate utilization of services and misuse of resources, and typically is not a criminal or intentional act" [3]. Any health-care expenditure that the patient could go without and still not see a reduction in the quality of their care constitutes waste. The Institute of Medicine's report *The Healthcare Imperative: Lowering Costs and Improving Outcomes* concludes that of the 2.5 trillion dollars spent on health care in 2009, consumers wasted 765 billion dollars on things like unnecessary services, excessive administrative costs, overpriced goods and services, missed opportunities for prevention, and inefficiently delivered services [4]. The Dartmouth Institute for Health Policy concludes that approximately 30% of Medicaid clinical care spending could be eliminated without a material drop in the quality of outcomes [5].

Even though waste may not be intentional, it can result in significant penalties for those who engage in it. The Centers for Medicare & Medicaid Services (CMS), insurance companies, and patients are all victims of waste by health-care professionals. When they find out about it, they take action to redress it, which can have dire consequences for a provider, as we will explore later on in this chapter. In addition to the direct consequences waste can have upon you and your practice, the increased cost created by wasteful health-care practices adds significantly to the crippling cost of health care in the USA. In fact, according to the White House, "slowing the growth rate of health care costs will prevent disastrous increases in the federal budget deficit ..., lower the unemployment rate consistent with steady inflation, ... and improve the standard of living by improving efficiency" [6]. Stopping the spread of waste in health care can not only save you from potential reputational and economic ruin, if the government is correct, but it will also go a long way toward saving the entire country from a similar fate.

Abuse

Like fraud, abuse takes on several different definitions. In general, though, a health-care provider commits abuse when they engage in conduct that diverges in a material way from sound, commonly accepted practices. An abusive behavior can involve not only questionable dental conduct but also aberrant business or fiscal practices.

As they do with respect to fraud, federal regulations provide a clear definition for the term abuse with respect to Medicare and Medicaid. According to Medicaid Program Integrity regulations, abuse results when a provider engages in "provider practices that are inconsistent with sound fiscal, business, or medical practices, and result in an unnecessary cost to the Medicaid program, or in reimbursement for services that are not medically necessary or that fail to meet professionally recognized standards for health care. It also includes beneficiary practices that result in unnecessary cost to the Medicaid program" [7]. The Medicare Program Integrity Manual is considerably less wordy. It characterizes abuse as "Billing Medicare for services that are not covered or are not correctly coded" [8].

Each of these definitions makes clear that abuse, unlike fraud, does not require intentional deceit. Abuse simply requires that a dentist do something that the reasonably prudent dentist would not do, most commonly with respect to acquire payment from a third party. For many providers, the lack of any requirement for intentional deceit likely makes abusive behaviors even easier to rationalize. Do not be fooled. While the penalties will likely be stricter if you commit intentional fraud, abuse can land you in hot water just as quickly with patients, with CMS, and with insurance companies. To commit fraud, waste, or abuse can derail even the most promising dental career.

Bad behavior

Now that we have determined what the terms fraud, waste, and abuse mean, let's take a look at some of the most common examples. We will talk about what each of these behaviors is, how to identify it, and what makes it fraudulent, wasteful, or abusive.

Bill for services not rendered

Billing for services not rendered presents, likely, the most egregiously fraudulent conduct on the entire continuum of fraud, waste, and abuse. You will likely (hopefully!) scoff at the idea of submitting a claim or bill to a payer for a service that you didn't provide. In the classic case, a bad actor simply fabricates a line item on a bill or claim where it is hard for anyone with even a shred of integrity to fathom billing for services not rendered. A clearer instance of dental fraud is difficult to imagine.

On the other hand, however, at least two other ways exist for a dentist to wind up in trouble for billing for services not rendered. In one case, you may not even have done anything wrong, but either way, the result will be the same. You will be held accountable for not providing the services you claim to have provided.

Right a wrong

As you have likely experienced firsthand, a dentist who participates with insurance carriers or provides services for government programs often laments that these payers drastically reduce the fees a provider can collect. Where a dentist might charge $1000 for a particular service, by virtue of participating in with an insurer's provider network, he might be limited to collect only $500 total for that service. Moreover, compared to the fee reductions of a commercial insurance program, government program reimbursement can make a dentist feel like the victim of highway robbery!

The reductions to fees to which a dentist agrees in order to participate in a given network can place the dentists into a precarious financial position, but they must fend off the temptation to "get it back" in other areas: to right a wrong. Some dentists, it seems, cannot resist the temptation to right a wrong. Frustrated by the fees they receive, they rationalize adding services to their dental claims in order to recoup what they feel the third-party payer has taken from them. They feel that their actions somehow right a wrong. Nothing could be further from the truth. No matter how one might rationalize it, consciously billing for a service not rendered is fraud.

You must avoid falling into this persecution complex. The simple fact that your agreement with an insurance company or government gives you lower reimbursement than your standard rate does not entitle you to create additional charges to recoup what has been "taken from you." At the risk of sounding unduly harsh, you must realize that nobody owes you anything. The truth is that you made an agreement to take those lower fees when you signed up with that insurance company or when you agreed to perform services to participate in that government program. Some benefit(s) you thought you would receive (access to more patients, in most cases) led you to agree to the detriment of reduced fees. In theory, at least, you made your decision to participate in these networks with eyes wide open. If you can't make your business model work given the fees you agree to accept, you likely need to reexamine whether your continued participation in these programs provides you with the benefit you anticipated when you first joined.

Undocumented treatment

Another way that providers find themselves on the wrong side of an allegation that they billed for services not rendered comes when an auditor finds a claim and a charge for services, but does not find corresponding entries in the patient's dental record at the dentist's office.

Both government programs and commercial insurers reserve the right to audit provider records. These audits allow the government and carriers to confirm that the dentists actually performed the treatments for which the payers paid them. If these payers cannot confirm the performance of the claimed service, they will seek recovery of any amounts paid, regardless of whether the dentist actually performed the service. The burden is on the provider to show that he performed the service. If the patient's dental record does not support the payment, that proof will make for a very steep uphill climb.

Similarly, even where a record exists, it may not provide sufficient evidence to allow the dentist to receive payment. Third-party payers consistently condition their payments on the existence of certain factors. Some of those factors include the requirement that the procedure be dentally necessary, that a treatment has not been provided within a certain amount of time prior to the procedure, that another condition exists, or that certain other measures were taken prior to resorting to the chosen treatment. Regardless of whether the program conditions its payment on dental necessity or some other factor, if the payer audits the dentist, the dentist must substantiate that the treatment met the requisite condition for payment. Whether the auditor is with CMS or with an insurance carrier, he will look at a treatment that he cannot substantiate as a treatment that was not performed and thus recover any payment made for that service. Sure, you very well may have done that restoration. There is a filling in the tooth, after all. But if there is no treatment note to indicate that you did it; there is no pre- and postoperative radiograph to show when, where, or by whom the filling was performed; and you can't prove that you did it, you will be paying the insurer back.

Unlike the case in which a dentist fabricates a treatment out of whole cloth and then adds it to his billing or claim form, this undocumented treatment does not necessarily constitute fraud. A dentist may fall victim to his own poor record keeping and in the process cost himself a significant sum of money.

Recovery of amounts for services not substantiated by patient dental records may seem harsh where a dentist knows that he performed the service. However, when a dentist performs a treatment without proper documentation, he commits abuse and contributes to waste within the health-care system. Imagine if dentists were not required to have records that substantiated their treatment. How would a payer ever verify the treatments he/she paid for? How would a subsequent treating dentist ever confirm a patient's history? Obviously, they couldn't. Both of these circumstances create the opportunity for providers to receive payment for work they never did, and both would necessarily lead to wasteful spending as new providers undertake needless examinations, radiographs, and other diagnostic measures to determine what would already be apparent had the initial provider properly documented his treatment.

Unnecessary service

Billing for unnecessary procedures stems from two types of cases. In the first case, a provider knows a procedure is not necessary, but performs it and bills for it in order to generate additional revenue. One example of billing for an unnecessary service might occur when a provider performs a filling in an intact tooth. Yes, he drilled and filled the tooth, so it is not a misrepresentation to say that he did so. However, if the tooth didn't need it, the procedure still should not have been done and constitutes fraud. In the second type of case, the provider believes he needs to perform the procedure (whether of his own volition or at the insistence of his patient) when, in fact, the patient does not need it. An example of this sort of behavior comes when a provider performs a crown on a tooth that really only needs a filling, "just to be safe."

In the first case, the provider shows the requisite intent for the procedure to constitute fraud. In fact, the provider not only engages in fraud but also likely malpractice and potentially criminal activity. The provider in the second case does not commit fraud, but still engages in abuse by performing a service that the reasonable and prudent dentist in his position would not perform: one that costs the patient and the public or private insurer money that they should not have to spend.

As with billing for services not rendered, dentists may try to rationalize their performance of unnecessary procedures, and these rationalizations ring just as hollow. It is easy, for instance, for a practitioner to believe that providing an unnecessary radiograph, sealant, or even periodontal treatment does no harm and doesn't cost the patient money. What the provider fails to consider, though, is that those procedures do have a cost and, furthermore, that to perform a procedure on a patient who doesn't need it, they engage in both waste and abuse while completely abusing the patient's trust.

Unbundle

A provider engages in "unbundling" when, instead of billing for a particular procedure code, he breaks the procedure down into its component parts and bills for each of the parts separately in order to receive a greater fee. For instance, when performing a three-surface restoration on a single posterior tooth, a dentist might attempt to charge for three single-surface restorations along with the anesthesia, adhesive, etching, liner, base, pulp cap, polish, occlusal adjustment, and caries removal. The resin-based composite—three-surface—posterior code is inclusive of all the separate procedures. To bill independently for each of them in addition to the base code constitutes double dipping. The same can be said when a provider bills for procedures for customization of a crown that are normally in all crowns like shading the crown to match existing dentition and building in an anatomic form.

To bill for each component part of a service separately results in a higher fee for the dentist. However, commercial and government payers have strict rules against unbundling. Before agreeing to participate in a commercial or government payer's network, be sure that you know the rules applicable to their participating providers.

Upcode

Upcode occurs when a provider performs a service and submits a code that reflects a procedure that is similar to the one provided but pays a higher amount. Upcoding most often falls into the category of fraud. Those who commit the offense do so with the knowledge that the code they submit does not correspond to the service they performed, and the intent is to collect more money than they would have collected had they submitted the proper code. One common example comes when a provider performs an extraction, erupted tooth or exposed root, but instead submits a claim for the surgical removal of erupted tooth requiring elevation of mucoperiosteal flap and removal of bone and/or section of the tooth. The surgical extraction invariably pays more money than does the extraction, and only a thin line exists between the two procedures. So some dentists have little or no trouble submitting for a surgical extraction instead of an extraction even when they well know what they performed.

In rare instances, however, to upcode constitutes abuse rather than fraud. In such cases, a provider merely mischaracterizes the service as something more complex or difficult than performed. Such a case might include a dentist honestly coding for an extraction when an extraction of coronal remnants was performed. The fact that the dentist has no malice and didn't intend to defraud does not make the upcode any more correct.

An ethical dentist must avoid the pull to upcode. It does not matter whether there is intent to defraud a payer or a simple application of the improper code for a procedure. Dentists who code for a more expensive procedure than the one performed betray the trust of their patients and their profession and end up paying for it financially, with a hit to their reputation, or both.

Kickback

Unlike some businesses, medical professionals cannot provide a "kickback" for referral or steering of patients to their office. A kickback occurs when a dental provider pays a person to refer people to their practice to receive dental services. While such practices commonly occur in other fields, such as real estate and retail, federal law prohibits them in the medical arena, including dental care, at least where the goods or services are provided under a federal health-care program such as Medicaid.

But what makes kickbacks verboten? What is wrong with referrals? They may lead to several abusive—potentially fraudulent—behaviors. For instance, if a dentist offers a referral fee to another dentist to refer patients to him for root canal therapy, those patients will likely receive root canal therapy whether they need it or not. Given these incentives, dentists let their decision making be altered by thoughts, ideas, and drivers other than the patient's medical need. In turn, these artificial incentives not only drive overutilization, but they also increase the costs paid by federal health-care programs and pervert the market for dental services. We will discuss the details of the federal Anti-Kickback Statute later on in this chapter.

Altered date of service

Dishonest dental providers in search of additional revenue often alter the date of service on which they provide treatment in order to maximize the benefits available to their patients. Such behavior constitutes clear fraud, as a provider or his staff must willfully do something dishonest (report an incorrect date of service) in order to acquire some added and undeserved benefit (reimbursement from a third-party payer).

To alter a date of service matters because many dental services paid for by an insurance plan have frequency limitations that set the number of times the insurance company will pay for a given service over a given amount of time. For instance, insurance plans commonly benefit an adult prophylaxis twice in a calendar year. If a patient comes in for a prophylaxis on January 3, July 5, and December 20, that makes three prophylaxis treatments in 1 year, and the insurer will not pay for the December 20 prophylaxis due to frequency limitations. A provider holds that December 20 claim until after January 1st or the New Year before submitting it with a date of service sometime in the New Year. That way, the frequency limitation has been reset, and the insurer will pay the claim. The prophylaxis is paid at 100%, so the patient receives a service with no out-of-pocket expense: no harm, no foul. Except it's fraud whether the alteration of the treatment date is at the behest of the patient or initiated by the dentist.

Discount

Even the most honest dentist commonly has a hard time understanding what is wrong with discounting a fee to a patient. If done correctly, nothing is wrong with it. To allow the patient to pay less money than would normally be paid or less than the dentist would normally charge another patient sounds like generosity, not fraud, waste, or abuse. In some cases, the discount is a generous gesture. In other cases, however, to provide a discount to the patient while still charging the insurer the full fee constitutes fraud or abuse.

The coinsurance provisions of dental benefit plans require dental insurance carriers to pay a percentage of the amount allowed to the provider and the patient to pay the rest. For instance, in a plan with 20% coinsurance, if a provider charges his patient $100 for a service, the insurance carrier must pay $80, while the patient must pay 20% of the allowed amount, or $20. It seems like a generous way to give the patient a financial break when a provider waives the patient's portion of the charge while the provider collects a reasonable amount for the service, an amount the insurance carrier already expected to pay.

However, writing off the patient's coinsurance through a discount really enables the provider and patient to defraud the insurance company into bearing a disproportionate share of the cost of care. After all, the insurance company agreed to pay 80% of the amount the provider is allowed to charge. By writing off the patient's $20 portion while still collecting the full $80 from the insurer, the provider makes clear that he really only intends to collect $80. Therefore, the insurance company's share of the payment should be 80% of $80, or $64. The patient should be expected to pay the $16 balance.

In instances where the patient truly cannot pay their full share, many dental insurance carriers have a method to allow providers to write off portion of the fee. In most cases, at a minimum, this requires the provider to request permission to do the write-off. The carrier does not require the provider to get its permission simply because it wants to make the provider's life difficult.

The carrier requires such permission in order to keep the write-offs from going unnoticed and distort the insurance market. As many states have recognized, the routine waiver of patients' share of insurance payments removes "the incentive that copayments and deductibles create in making the consumer a cost-conscious purchaser of health care" [9]. That is, if a patient doesn't have to worry about paying for a health-care service, he doesn't really have to consider whether that treatment is necessary or helps him toward a better outcome. This distortion of consumer motivations leads to waste and higher health-care costs by forcing insurers and other third-party payers to pay for services that patients don't really need, when they could have used those same funds to pay for truly necessary goods and services. Insurers then pass these increased costs back to the market in the form of higher premiums and lower payouts on legitimate claims.

Who's looking?

Now that we have detailed the many avenues a provider might take to engage in fraud, waste, or abuse, we need to examine the very real possibility of getting caught. More importantly, we'll also look at the consequences a dentist could face if he does get caught. Think of this section as our dental version of *Scared Straight!* Instead of convicted felons scaring unwitting teenagers onto the right path in order to avoid the convicts' plight, though, you'll have to settle for a health-care lawyer relaying the perils that await dentists who attempt to cheat the system.

As well-educated experts in your chosen field, it might occur to you that you have enough of a knowledge advantage over your patients that you could get away with telling them just about anything. That is not to say that most dentists *would* try to get away with such a thing. However, one cannot deny that a natural disparity of information exists between dental professionals and their patients. How many patients have the oral health knowledge to challenge your diagnosis of an infected nerve requiring a root canal as opposed to a toothache caused by a simple case of caries that may only require a simple filling? How many patients have the wherewithal to contest your diagnosis of the need for a crown rather than a two-surface filling? Not too many. Please don't be fooled, however. You may be surprised to learn just how many different constituencies are actually out there keeping track of your behavior and ready to hold you accountable. If and when they do, you will find a variety of consequences that will impact you in a variety of ways, from damaging your reputation to costing you money to keeping you from practicing your chosen profession to potentially even taking away your freedom.

First, although I just spent an entire paragraph assuring you that *most* of your patients won't have the knowledge or gumption to challenge your treatment decisions or your billing practices, rest assured that patients do exist who would like nothing more than to catch you lying to them and make your life miserable getting even. These individuals can hurt you in several ways: They can damage your reputation by talking to others about your unethical conduct. And remember, in this digital age, they are not just talking to their immediate friends and neighbors. Online forums exist for discussion and rating of dentists, as do accrediting organizations, such as the Better Business Bureau, and governmental entities charged with consumer protection such as the state attorney general's office, which exist solely to identify, catalogue, investigate, and potentially rectify consumer issues. Even if no civil or criminal complaint arises, once an issue has been identified and reported, it will very likely have some lasting reputational impact.

Speaking of civil and criminal cases, I would be remiss if I did not identify an additional set of individuals with substantial motivation to identify your wrongdoing: lawyers. Lawyers stand to make a substantial amount of money holding you accountable for violations of the law. Specifically, qui tam lawyers have identified health-care fraud as a lucrative field to ply their trade. Qui tam lawyers specialize in bringing claims on behalf of the government pursuant to the False Claims Act. The False Claims Act is a federal law that allows the government to sue those individuals who attempt to defraud the government by making false claims for payment. The law contains a provision that allows members of the public who are aware of an attempt to defraud the government to bring a lawsuit against that person on the government's behalf. If the person who brings the suit, the "relator," wins the case, he or she will receive between 15 and 30% of the government's damages. Damages in a False Claims Act case can be enormous, too. The Act calls for penalties that range from $5500 per claim to $11,000 per claim [10].

So, if your office receives payment for its services from Medicaid, Medicare, Children's Health Insurance Program (CHIP), or any other federally funded program and your office submits a claim that it knows is fraudulent with the intent to collect more money for that claim than is actually owed, you might be liable for up to $11,000 plus three times the amount of the false claim. For example, if you submit a claim for a $1000 crown that you did not do, you could be liable under the False Claims Act for $14,000 for that one crown: $11,000 penalty, plus three times the $1000 false claim or $3000. That sounds like a lot for one claim, but it is even more mind-boggling when you think about systemic problems, such as always upcoding a certain kind of claim. If a dentist upcodes every standard extraction to a surgical extraction that costs $1500 and the dentist submits 200 such extraction claims in a year, that dentist could be on the hook for $3,100,000. That is $1500 in damages per claim times three because of treble damages for a total of $4500 plus a possible $11,000 penalty per claim equals $15,500 per claim. Multiplied by 200 claims, the total liability would be $3,100,000. Now, the government might not impose the full penalty in every instance, and the damages may be reduced if the dentist can prove that part of the amount due was legitimate (i.e., a standard extraction was actually performed, so some part of the $1500 claimed to be due and owing may be taken into consideration). However, this example should illuminate the very real damages that can arise in one of these cases and underscore the incentive a qui tam plaintiff (and his attorney) would have to bring such an action. This heavy burden under the civil False Claims Act doesn't even take into account the potential criminal liability that can result under the federal criminal false claims statute, 18 USC § 287, which can result in fines of up to $250,000 and 5 years of imprisonment.

Qui tam attorneys are not the only third parties who can serve their own interests, as well as consumers', by exposing fraud waste and abuse by dentists. In fact, that is one of the most significant aspects of my job as a compliance director. That is, I look for fraud, waste, or abuse by providers, and I recover for my company's members who have overpaid, I recover for my company if it has overpaid, and I report to the government as well if we are administering the program for the government. In some cases, I even recommend the provider's termination from our company's network of providers. In those cases, it is not just the money lost from having to pay back for incorrect claims that hurts the provider. The inability to treat individuals who are insured by our company can continue to impact a dentist long after he compensated our company and the patient for the incorrect claim. In one recent instance, a provider that was terminated from our network actually sold his practice and gave up the practice of dentistry rather than trying to make it as a nonparticipating provider.

I mentioned government reporting in the preceding section, and I believe that topic deserves its own discussion here. When we discover wrongdoing by a provider, there are any number of different regulatory actors to whom we report that activity. The reporting requirements will vary from state to state. In this section, I will give a summary review of the reporting requirements to which we are subject in the state of Colorado, where I work.

First, if we determine it necessary to terminate a provider from our network for a reason associated with clinical ability to practice or take any action that adversely affects the ability to practice for more than 30 days, we must report it to the National Practitioner Data Bank. The data bank is a repository of information intended created by the federal government to facilitate the review of the professional credentials of health-care practitioners, entities, providers, and suppliers. Also, if we conclude that the action is fraudulent and seek to adjust a claim that is more than 1 year old, Colorado law requires us to report the fraud to the "appropriate law enforcement and regulatory entities in the investigation and prosecution of insurance fraud" [11]. Those reports go the Colorado Attorney General's Insurance Fraud Unit and the Colorado Division of Insurance. In cases where we settle a lawsuit or acquire a judgment against a provider, we report to those two entities, as well as the Colorado State Board of Dental Examiners pursuant to Colorado Division of Insurance Regulation 6-5-1. In Colorado, insurance fraud is a crime that ranges from a class 1 misdemeanor to a class 5 felony, which can include up to 2 years of jail time. In cases that involve the state Medicaid program, the fines and imprisonment are governed by federal false claims law, which, as detailed earlier, would allow up to $250,000 in fines ($500,000 for a corporation) and up to 5 years of imprisonment.

Reports to governmental authorities by patients, fellow practitioners, or insurance carriers such as those detailed earlier can certainly have significant negative implications to a provider's finances and his freedom. The impact a negative report can have, however, does not end with a fine or even a jail term. Both the state and federal government have means of impacting your ability to practice even after you've paid a fine or served a sentence. Each state has a licensing authority for dentists that serve as a gatekeeper to the practice of dentistry in that state. Upon receiving word of fraud, waste, or abuse by a provider, a state licensing board may elect to take disciplinary action up to and including the revocation of a dentist's license to practice in the state. In Colorado, for instance, the Dental Practice Act authorizes disciplinary action by the board when a provider engages in the "false billing in the delivery of dental or dental hygiene services, including, but not limited to, performing one service and billing for another, billing for any service not rendered, or committing a fraudulent insurance act." While the financial pain that can come from a fine or having to reimburse a patient or insurance company can undoubtedly sting, the inability to practice going forward into the future will have the longer-lasting impact.

Similarly, while the federal government does not license dentists, it can prohibit them from practicing and being reimbursed as part of any federally funded program. When a provider has an adverse outcome, including an instance of fraud, waste, or abuse, the Office of the Inspector General (OIG) can seek to exclude that provider from practicing as part of a federally funded program. Federally funded programs include Medicare, Medicaid, and CHIP. If the OIG determines that the person or entity must be prohibited from participating in a federal health-care program, the person's or entity's name is added to the OIG's List of Excluded Individuals and Entities (LEIE).

As federally funded health-care programs expand, appearing on the LEIE has enormous consequences that reach beyond the fact that the provider will not be allowed to receive any payments from any such program. Any entity contracting with the federal government or a state government administering a federally funded health-care program is also prohibited from employing or contracting with a person or entity that appears on the LEIE. With many states expanding their Medicaid programs to include dental, with Medicaid spending projected to increase by 6.8% per year through 2023, and with the Congress expected to reauthorize CHIP funding through at least 2019, these federally funded health-care programs will likely comprise an even greater slice of dental practitioners' business for the foreseeable future. To be excluded from participating in such programs will have a correspondingly larger impact.

Fraud, waste, and abuse in your office

We hope that you read the preceding sections of this chapter and thought, "I am never going to be tempted to engage in fraud, waste, or abuse. It's just not worth it! I could lose my license, my practice, my money, and my freedom." Perhaps the scariest part of this chapter, though, is that even if you personally never engage in fraud, waste, or abuse, the individuals you employ can put you at risk as well.

That's right, in nearly every case in which I identified fraud, waste, or abuse by a dentist, at some point, the dentists have blamed their staff:

"We had some staff that really didn't know what they were doing."

"I had an office manager who just couldn't remember the difference between simple extraction and a surgical extraction."

"We resubmitted every denied bitewing series as 4 periapical films? My assistant handles all of our claim submissions. I don't know how that happened."

"My hygienist didn't realize she couldn't submit a claim for work she did when I wasn't actually in the office to supervise her."

"We had an employee who was stealing from us. He was the one who submitted these claims. We're victims too."

You know what I tell them? It doesn't matter who clicked the button to submit the claim. You are responsible for the claims that are submitted with your name on them. Right there on the ADA-approved claim form, in a box marked "53," it states, "I hereby certify that the procedures as indicated by date are in progress (for procedures that require multiple visits) or have been completed."

Where I work, we use a form with slightly modified language. Our form states, "I hereby certify that I have performed the procedures as indicated by date and/or wish to predetermine the procedures which are not dated. the procedures were/are necessary in my professional judgment." Once your name is signed in that box, you are responsible for the submission. No ifs, ands, or buts about it.

The fact that someone else submitted it does not exonerate you or entitle you to keep money for claims submitted erroneously. Even if you can prove that you didn't have anything to do with the false claim submission and it really was the staff member's fault, that doesn't change the fact that money will be recovered for claims submitted incorrectly. By that time, you will have likely spent the money, and even having to pay it back will present a very real problem, to say nothing of potential fines and penalties that come from having submitted false claims.

How to avoid fraud, waste, and abuse

So how can you avoid fraud, waste, and abuse in your office? How can you ensure that you and your staff remain committed to do the right thing and perform only necessary treatment and submit claims only for the service actually performed? How can you ensure that your office stays committed even when the going gets tough? It will not likely come as a surprise to you that a guy like me, who makes his career as a compliance director, recommends implementing an effective compliance program.

If I seem biased, don't take it just from me; take it from the US Department of Health and Human Services OIG. The OIG offers the following five tips for creating a culture of compliance in the health-care workplace [12]:

1 Make compliance plans a priority now.
2 Know your fraud and abuse risk areas.

3 Manage your financial relationships.
4 Just because your competitor is doing something doesn't mean you can or should. Call 1-800-HHS-TIPS to report suspect practices.
5 When in doubt, ask for help.

Number 1 is first for a reason. The US Sentencing Commission's Guidelines Manual, which sets forth the federal sentencing guidelines, created dramatic incentives to implement an effective corporate compliance program. The federal sentencing guidelines are policies and practices promulgated by the US Sentencing Commission in accordance with the Sentencing Reform Act of 1984 [13]. These policies and practices provide guidance to judges charged with handing down criminal sentences to individuals as well as the entities they lead after they are convicted of crimes.

While a dental practice, like any company, cannot go to jail, it can be subjected to some hefty fines as detailed earlier. However, under the federal sentencing guidelines, an organization that has been convicted of a crime receives a culpability score that serves as a modifier to the sentence the organization will receive. An organization can reduce its "culpability score" by 3 points for having an effective compliance and ethics program. This could mean reducing any fines applicable to the company by more than 90%. For example, in a case where a company faces $1,000,000 "base fine" and has a culpability score of 3, the actual fine the company would pay would be a minimum of $600,000 [14]. With an effective compliance and ethics program, however, the federal sentencing guidelines would reduce the score to zero, and the fine could be limited to $50,000. That's a reduction of 91.6% just by having an effective compliance and ethics program!

To receive the benefit of that reduction, though, the compliance and ethics program must not only exist, but it must also be effective according to the guidelines. The federal sentencing guidelines set forth a minimum necessary set of requirements that render a compliance and ethics program effective for the purposes of decreasing a company's culpability score [15]. While they provide sound guidance for any organization that seeks to craft an effective compliance and ethics program, these standards do not readily avail themselves to application to small health-care practices.

Fortunately, the OIG published further guidance on the implementation of effective compliance programs in a wide variety of different businesses. The OIG created a more specific framework in which to build an effective compliance program for individual and small group physician practices. The same sort of program can easily apply to a dental practice. While expressly acknowledging that not every practice will have the financial and staffing resources to implement every facet of the program, the OIG sets forth the following seven "components of an effective compliance program" for individual and small group practices:

1 Conduct internal monitoring and auditing
   The first critical aspect that the OIG identifies for an effective compliance program is an ongoing evaluation process [16]. My experience with compliance programs bears out the OIG's recommendation. Without an ongoing

monitoring system, one cannot know whether the policies and standards in place at the practice accurately reflect the current law and provide an effective tool to aid in abiding by such law.

Conducting routine auditing and monitoring will allow the practice to ensure that the policies and practices are up to date and that by following them, the practice employees can be certain that so long as they abide by the policies and procedures, they will conduct themselves—and therefore conduct the practice—lawfully. Furthermore, even if the audit concludes that the policies and procedures reflect the current law and that the staff abides by them in conducting their business affairs, the audit will still likely aid the practice in identifying any areas of weakness. This will allow the dentists to act to mitigate the risks associated with the weaknesses before they become instances of noncompliance.

2   Implement compliance and practice standards

One might argue that the OIG put the cart before the horse with respect to recommending monitoring and auditing program to determine "whether the … practice's standards and procedures are in fact current and accurate" before it recommends implementing written standards and procedures. Nonetheless, the guidance does correctly point out the value of written standards and procedures in reducing the likelihood of fraudulent or otherwise aberrant behaviors. When people know exactly what they are supposed to do, the risk of them doing it wrong goes down dramatically. Seems pretty simple.

The OIG recommends having standards in place for four key risk areas. You will note that these key risk areas align closely with the areas of potential fraud, waste, and abuse detailed earlier in this chapter. The key risk areas the OIG identifies for the implementation of standards and procedures are (i) code and bill, (ii) reasonable and necessary services, (iii) documentation, and (iv) improper inducements, kickbacks, and referrals. Note that these four areas cover each and every "bad behavior" set forth earlier and several of the bad behaviors fall into more than one of the key risk areas:

- Code and bill—Bill for services not rendered, bill for unnecessary services, unbundle, upcode, alter the date of service, and discounting
- Reasonable and necessary services—Bill for unnecessary services, overutilization, and kickbacks
- Documentation—Bill for services not rendered, bill for unnecessary service, alter the date of service, and discounting
- Improper inducement, kickback, and referral—Bill for unnecessary services, kickbacks, and discounting

Record retention

In addition to standards and procedures necessary in these high-risk areas to prevent the bad behaviors, the OIG recommends that an effective compliance program for an individual or small group practice develops a standard schedule for record retention. In particular, the OIG notes, individual and small group practices would be wise to set up record retention policies for their compliance, business, and medical records.

Retaining the practice's compliance documents makes perfect sense. If a practice invests the time and money to enroll its members into educational programs, undertake internal investigations of issues that arise, and evaluate its own performance with audits and self-assessments, it stands to reason that the practice would want proof of its efforts if ever a regulator came calling. The same proof would come in handy in the event—however undesirable—that the practice looks to reduce a criminal sentence by way of an effective compliance program. Even absent the need to prove the efficacy of the practice's compliance program, the compliance documentation from educational programs, internal investigations, and audits will undoubtedly provide value in the future when the next similar issue arises.

3 Designate a compliance officer or contact

In order to have an effective individual or small group practice compliance program, you should designate a single person to act as the compliance officer or at least to serve as the primary compliance contact for each issue or type of issue that arises. As the OIG notes, this designation can take many forms.

In the event that a dental practice designates a single person to oversee all compliance activities, they should have several key duties. First, the compliance designee oversees and monitors the implementation of the compliance program. The practice's compliance professional establishes methods to improve the practice's efficiency and reduce its susceptibility to fraud, waste, and abuse. When the law or the practice's compliance needs change, the designated compliance person takes it upon themselves to become aware of the change and address it for the practice. The compliance person should also develop and implement a compliance training program, ensure that the LEIE is cross-checked regularly against the practice's employees and contractors, and investigate any report or allegation concerning improper conduct by practice employees.

This list makes clear, to me, why designating one or more people to address compliance activities has so much value compared to designating a person to address each issue as it arises. Rather than wait for an issue to present itself by way of a deficiency or wait to find a weakness during a self-audit that needs to be cured, designate a person(s) ahead of time who is responsible for each of the duties set forth earlier so that you have a proactive compliance program instead of a reactionary one.

To have a designated leader focus on potential compliance issues and addresses them before they arise enables you to keep your compliance program on the cutting edge and truly effective. As we know by now, an effective compliance program serves as a real asset in the event that the practice faces sentencing for a conviction. More importantly, an effective compliance program will likely keep you from ever having to worry about a conviction in the first place.

4 Conduct effective training and education

An effective compliance program directs training to the specific needs of the practice without ignoring indispensable general compliance training. In order for training to accomplish those dual goals, the dental practice must plan accordingly. In order to provide effective training, a dental practice must first determine who will arrange the training. Regardless of whether the practice designates a compliance officer who handles training or selects an individual to manage the training, three things need to be determined: (i) who needs training, (ii) what style of training work bests, and (iii) when and how often should training take place.

No two compliance training programs look exactly alike. However, in order to be effective, each must answer the three questions set forth earlier, and they must do so in furtherance of the two primary goals of compliance training. As the OIG notes, the two primary goals of compliance training must be to ensure (i) that all employees understand how to perform their jobs in compliance with the rules, regulations, and other standards applicable to them and (ii) that all employees understand that they must continue to comply with these obligations for as long as they remain employed with the practice. While annual compliance training is most often sufficient to address the second goal, a single one-size-fits-all training will not likely suffice to ensure that all employees understand how to perform their jobs in compliance with the rules applicable to them. Therefore, every effective compliance program has general compliance training at least annually, and most require more detailed job-specific training on top of that.

Regardless of whether a practice conducts only annual training or has compliance training for each department on a regular basis, the goals remain the same. First, all employees in a dental office must know and abide by the rules, regulations, statutes, laws, and other standards that apply to them. Second, employees must also understand that to abide to the provisions of the compliance program will not get the employee into trouble, while failure to comply will result in some form of discipline, up to and including termination.

5 Respond appropriately to detected offenses and develop corrective action

Detecting noncompliance is only half the battle. If the practice never takes steps to correct the problem it identifies, it doesn't really help the practice to avoid fraud, waste, or abuse. A compliance program cannot truly have a positive effect on the practice unless it appropriately addresses the compliance issues it identifies.

Fraud, waste, and abuse come in all shapes and sizes. Consequently, so should your response when you identify an instance of noncompliance. Indeed, your practice need not respond to every failure to comply with a rule or law by firing the whole staff and start from scratch. On the other hand, no one improves when you fail to ever take any action in response to noncompliance.

But how do you determine the proper response to a violation of rule, law, or other compliance standard? First, your practice performs a full assessment of any report of noncompliance. This helps you to determine where noncompliant behavior falls related to the standards and procedures your program has in place. Is it a violation that toes the line between compliant and noncompliant, or is it a flagrant violation? In addition to help determine the severity of the compliance violation, a full assessment of the reported violation also helps determine how the violation occurred. Was it the result of your compliance program's inability to detect noncompliant behavior—which requires modification of the compliance plan in order to detect future instances before they occur? Was it a coordinated effort by the violator or violators to circumvent the compliance program?

When determining the appropriate response to violations that occur—and they will occur—you must evaluate each instance of noncompliance individually. Even when two violations of the same type occur, such as when a dentist submits an insurance claim for a surgical extraction instead of the more appropriate extraction, the pertinent facts and circumstances may dictate vastly different corrective actions. The two cases have the same result (upcode an extraction to a surgical one), but one may be the innocent mistake of a staffer who read the dentist's clinical note incorrectly, while in the other case the clinical note is blatantly and fraudulently amended when he knew without question what it should have been coded. Both cases clearly involve noncompliant behaviors. However, in the former instance, perhaps some coding training is in order for the claim submission staff, and some training with respect to complete, adequate, and clear treatment notes makes sense for the dentists. The latter case, on the other hand, is clear fraud and warrants strict discipline and potentially termination.

6 Develop open lines of communication

Open, effective communication must exist in order to have an effective compliance program. Without it, employees may not know how or may not feel comfortable reporting instances of suspected noncompliance. This deprives your practice of its primary source to learn about instances of noncompliant fraudulent, wasteful, or abusive conduct. In order to ensure that this open and effective communication exists, you must ensure that employees know that the terms of their employment require them to report any conduct that a reasonable person would believe to be fraudulent, wasteful, abusive, or otherwise outside of established standards of conduct.

To facilitate this open and effective communication, the OIG recommends implementing several important items [17]:

- User-friendly process such as anonymous drop box
- Provision in the practice's standards and procedures that state that the failure to report erroneous or fraudulent conduct violates the compliance program
- Simple and readily accessible procedure for processing reports of erroneous or fraudulent behavior
- Process to maintain the anonymity of both the person involved in the potentially erroneous or fraudulent behavior being reported and the person reporting such conduct

- Provision in the practice's standards and procedures that prohibit retribution, retaliation, or any adverse employment consequences resulting from a good faith report of what the reporting party believes to be fraudulent, wasteful, abusive, or otherwise noncompliant behavior

  To implement a communication system like that detailed earlier ensures that all members of your dental practice not only know what they must report but also how to report it and—just as importantly—that they will not face an adverse consequence for making such a report in good faith.

7 Enforce standards through well-publicized disciplinary guidelines

In order to have a truly effective compliance program, the parties subject to that program must understand the potential outcomes if they violate the terms of the program [18]. If, for instance, a hygienist doesn't understand that they can be terminated when they fail to report a dentist in the practice who upcodes treatments, they may be less inclined to report the dentist's behavior.

Your practice must provide enough detail in its training and conduct materials so that all employees understand their responsibilities and the potential outcomes that might befall them if they fail to live up to those responsibilities. The trick to implement and enforce this disciplinary standard is to ensure that the practice applies the standard consistently and appropriately while also leaving enough flexibility to address the many facts and circumstances that can mitigate or aggravate the consequences necessary in a given situation.

To implement the OIG's seven elements of an effective compliance program, you will make your practice less susceptible to noncompliant behavior and also be well positioned, practically and legally, in the event that noncompliant behavior ever arises. Not only will your practice be readily able to address any fraud, waste, or abuse that occurs, but it will have the strength of the federal sentencing guidelines to mitigate any penalties that might follow from those behaviors.

Conclusion

Clearly, many avenues exist that can lead to trouble for dentists. A provider's greed can lead to any number of fraudulent behaviors in a misguided attempt to increase income, or inattention to important technicalities can result in a provider or her staff committing waste or abuse in the health-care system. Whatever road to misconduct a provider takes, the consequences of engaging in fraud, waste, or abuse can devastate a dentist's reputation, her financial well-being, and even her freedom. Don't let it happen to you.

In this chapter, we have explored several different types of fraud, waste, and abuse in which a provider might engage. We looked at billing for services not rendered, undocumented treatments, unnecessary services, unbundling, upcoding, kickbacks, altering dates of service, and discounting. Each area, whether intentional or not, can lead to dramatic consequences if identified in a dentist's practice.

Because we know that some incentive exists to engage in these behaviors despite their impropriety, we next delved into all of the ways in which a person engaged in fraud, waste, or abuse is likely to be caught. We have identified all those who might have an interest in bringing such a provider's scheme to an end and the consequences that will befall him if he's caught and apprehended. Hopefully, those consequences and the myriad ways in which a system of fraud, waste, or abuse can be identified and brought to justice provided you with the disincentive to keep you from engaging in it to begin with.

As we noted, however, even if you have no intention of engaging in fraud, waste, or abuse, you can fall victim to it if you do not proactively guard against it. For that reason, we introduced you to the value of implementing an effective compliance program to keep not only yourself but also your staff compliant with applicable laws and away from the pitfalls of fraudulent, wasteful, and/or abusive behaviors. While implementing an effective compliance program might seem daunting given its seven particular elements, the costs such a program can save by avoiding enforcement actions and the fines and penalties that follow from them make a compliance program indispensable. Moving forward, it appears the average health-care practitioner will see the cost of compliance more and more widely as simply a cost of doing business, much like insurance or electricity. In fact, in 2014, the *Wall Street Journal* called compliance officer "the hottest job in America" with both the number of jobs and salaries increasing dramatically in the past 10 years [19]. Membership in the Health Care Compliance Association, a health-care compliance industry trade group, has grown at a rate of 9% per year over the past 5 years [20]. Given the dramatic increase in regulation under the Affordable Care Act and the focus the federal government has placed upon increasing enforcement actions and to reducing health-care fraud, waste, and abuse, it is not hard to see why. Even the upstanding providers need someone to help them stay outta trouble.

References

1 Merriam-Webster.com. Fraud. September 23, 2014. http://www.merriam-webster.com/dictionary/fraud (accessed December 1, 2014).

2 The $272 billion swindle: why thieves love America's health-care system http://www.economist.com/news/united-states/21603078-why-thieves-love-americas-health-care-system-272-billion-swindle (accessed December 1, 2014).

3 National Association of Medicaid Directors. Rethinking medicaid program integrity: eliminating duplication and investing in effective, high-value tools. (2012, March), p. 4.

4 The cost of health care. http://resources.iom.edu/widgets/vsrt/healthcare-waste.html (accessed December 30, 2014).

5 Health Policy Briefs. Reducing waste in health care. http://www.healthaffairs.org/healthpolicybriefs/brief.php?brief_id=82 (accessed December 1, 2014).

6 The economic case for health care reform. http://www.whitehouse.gov/administration/eop/cea/TheEconomicCaseforHealthCareReform/ (accessed December 30, 2014).

7 42 U.S.C. § 455.2

8 Medicare Program Integrity Manual at Exhibit 1.

9 Colo. Rev. Stat. § 18-13-119(1)(b) (2014).

10 31 U.S.C. § 3729(a)(1); 28 CFR § 85.3(a)(9).

11 C.R.S. §§10-16-704(4.5)(m) and 10-1-128(5)(a)(IV).

12 Health Care Compliance Program Tips. https://oig.hhs.gov/compliance/provider-com pliance-training/files/Compliance101tips508.pdf (accessed December 30, 2014).

13 United States Sentencing Commission. *Guidelines manual, Part A* (2013).

14 United States Sentencing Commission. *Guidelines manual*, §§ 8B2.1, 8C2.5 (2013)

15 United States Sentencing Commission. *Guidelines manual*, § 8B2.1(b) (2013).

16 *Federal register*, Vol. 65, No. 194, Thursday, October 5, 2000 at 59437.

17 *Federal register*, Vol. 65, No. 194, Thursday, October 5, 2000 at 59444.

18 *Federal register*, Vol. 65, No. 194, Thursday, October 5, 2000 at 59434.

19 Compliance officer: dream career? As fines sting, a hiring spree for risk and compliance staff.   http://www.wsj.com/articles/SB10001424052702303330204579250722114538750 (accessed December 30, 2014).

20 Businesses hire up to deal with more regs. http://thehill.com/regulation/business/189770-businesses-hire-up-to-deal-with-mounting-regulations (accessed December 30, 2014).

CHAPTER 9

Analysis to action

Michael M. Okuji
Delta Dental of Colorado, Denver, USA

Introduction

This chapter suggests competitive strategies for subsets of the dental care delivery system. The suggested strategies are based on what we know, where we are, and where we want to go. Innovative strategy means to look outside of where we live today and venture to where we want to be tomorrow. To remain stagnant or on the sideline is to become irrelevant. All parts of the dental care delivery systems strive to deliver the appropriate service in the right amount, at the right time, where it is needed, to the right people at a lower cost. Innovative strategy marshals the available resources into new configurations. It doesn't just tinker with the existing model. Small private practice, group practice, group practice system, safety net system (SNS), and organized dentistry are examined to suggest competitive strategies. The dental industry and dental education are critical segments for the system as a whole but are not addressed here.

The goal is to suggest competitive strategies for each segment that are feasible, meaningful, sustainable, profitable, and actionable within the current legal framework and fiscal constraints. Innovative strategy to improve the dental care delivery system is critical because in the next decade more individuals will have access (financial and geographic) to dental care. And at its best, US dental care is the best in the world.

Premise

The premise is that the oral health-care delivery system is flawed in that it is inefficient to deliver appropriate care, in the appropriate amount, at the appropriate time, to the appropriate population, at an appropriate cost. The best of US dental care is limited to those with employer-based dental benefits.

The premise is that the current oral health-care delivery system does not and will not drive dental care delivery innovation because of ingrained satisfaction

Dental Benefits and Practice Management: A Guide for Successful Practices, First Edition.
Edited by Michael M. Okuji.
© 2016 John Wiley & Sons, Inc. Published 2016 by John Wiley & Sons, Inc.

with the status quo. Competitive strategy and innovation require an integrator of systems to step forward to integrate the system of dental care across functional silos. The integrator may not be a dentist. The current role of organized dentistry is to preserve professional autonomy and the practitioner's belief that dental care decisions are solely in their hands. This role changes as organized dentistry steps up to assume a different role as the integrator of individual dental practices. The role of the group system, the corporate practice of dentistry, is to support the current dental care system. This too changes when dental service organizations begin to fully leverage their presence to integrate horizontally and vertically. The role of the SNS, including federally qualified health centers, shifts as the dental portion of the Affordable Care Act (ACA) encompasses more individuals and becomes a robust program. Consumers will have choices other than the safety net clinic for their dental care. The dental portion of SNS is an important part of any community, but it requires an integrator to make them sustainable, productive, and profitable. And finally, the relationship of dental education with the community morphs as its dentists begin to assume different roles in the delivery of dental care.

The premise is that a vigorous (the will), robust (financial heft) integrator will step forward from one or multiple stakeholders to assemble the components of the current dental care delivery system, dismantle the silos and walls, and craft them into an innovative new system that is patient centered and outcome driven.

Competition

Competition in dental care delivery has important benefits for price, access, and health outcome. Many aspects of the ACA like transparency, accountability, payment models, revenue constraints, and the integration of dental care delivery, both horizontal and vertical, encourage innovation that ratchets up competition among the current segments of the system and invites new players.

One aspect of the competition is price competition. A lower cost of care broadens the access to dental care with the promise of better dental health outcomes. Price competition forces the players in dental care delivery to look at their cost to do business, spread the operating and capital expense over a wider footprint, and introduce operations efficiency in order to be competitive. This is a good thing.

Nonprice competition promotes innovation in a patient-centered practice that increases geographic access to care when and where it is needed, information on their care that is understandable, measurable satisfaction, positive outcome, and the maintenance of trust with the perception of ethical behavior from their dentist.

Competition can be unpleasant for the competitor and creates cognitive dissonance for some dentists. But competition inspires dentists to evaluate their business model and take action. In this sense, competition promotes the Triple Aim to deliver cost-efficient care of demonstrable quality that a patient values.

Information

Competition and innovative systems can't deliver on their promise without good information and properly aligned payment incentives. Competition doesn't eliminate the uncertainty in dental care or the asymmetry of information available to the consumers. Indeed, asymmetrical information limits competitive effectiveness. So competition and innovation require that consumers have access to understandable information about the price and quality of dental care. Today, it is difficult to get information about the price and quality of health-care services. Dental fees aren't publicly posted and quality benchmarks are not available. Some dental care entities are experimenting with quality metrics, report cards, and other strategies to disseminate information to consumers. Good information about the cost and quality of a dental service that is readily accessible is a critical competitive advantage.

Small private practice

The competitive strategy for the small private practice is to control what you can control. Streamline your practice to the nth degree that includes the administrative processes to make you more productive and patient centered. Begin to think in terms of margins and not averages, and expense control rather than increased fees. Partner with a colleague even if it's to share a new Panorex machine.

The solo private practice is the predominant model of dental practice and has remained pretty much unchanged in my 40-year private practice career: choose a location; find a lender; purchase equipment; hire staff; decide services to offer; ask a colleague for a fee list; set office hours; open the door; and it's autopilot for the next 40 years. It's all about me and how I want to work. That's why I picked dentistry as a profession.

But private practice is under siege. Dentist income is caught between rising operating costs that butt up against a revenue ceiling. Between 1980 and 2000, my productive years, the steep upward slope of dentist's income forgave imprudent decisions and fiscal mismanagement.

When revenue increased year after year, dentists had the luxury to establish and run their solo practice designed to satisfy their personal preferences. This meant their flexibility to set the location and size of a practice, number of hours worked, number of auxiliaries employed, cutting-edge equipment purchased (most ending up stored in the garage), and the mix of dental services offered was at the sole discretion of the dentist without regard to the larger economy, operational efficiency, and customer preferences. The year-over-year revenue increase shielded the dentist from financial misjudgment and masked financial waste. It seems that money covered a multitude of sins. Build it and they will come. This is the world in which I practiced.

But dental income and the number of patient visits have remained flat since 2000. This trend preceded the 2008 recession continues today. Dental plan fee allowances and maximums are static too. It appears as those trends will continue into the foreseeable future and no longer will increased fees mask operating waste and inefficiency. For a dentist to offset low fees by increasing the number of procedures per patient (intensity without necessity) to compensate for their flat revenue smacks of fraud, waste, and abuse, particularly abuse of their patient's trust.

A losing competitive strategy for the small private practice is to compete for the phantom fee-for-service all-cash patient who is willing and able to pay whatever fee the dentist decides to charge for quality practice. A losing strategy is the boutique practice that offers massage, manicure, and limousine service. A losing strategy is the botulinum and dermal fill cosmetic dental practice. A losing strategy is the concierge practice that smacks of elitism. These strategies target a sliver of the population and ignore the social covenant.

But there is a place for the small private practice to continue to thrive and deliver on the promise of patient-centered dental care. What does a solo dentist do to remain competitive? First, there are a number of steps that a small practice can take today. The steps revolve around the streamlined practice, patient-centered care, and process management to support efficiencies in care and cost and to think in terms of margin, not average.

Streamline

To streamline the small dental practice means to first take the easy first baby steps. Take baby steps today; don't wait for tomorrow. These steps prod you to think in terms of administrative (process) management. These steps are entirely in your control. Change the things you can change.

A baby step means that you implement processes to efficiently capture and deliver information and improve your cash flow—a dollar today is worth more than a dollar tomorrow. Easy baby steps are electronic predetermination of treatment, electronic insurance claim submission, and direct deposit. These steps break through the bottleneck in cash flow. These systems capture accurate information internally and disseminate externally to your patient—streamlined and patient centered in a single process.

Electronic eligibility of the patient can be done through the benefit company's website or interactive voice response (IVR) system. Patients generally know the name of their dental benefit carrier but little else. This is the fastest and most efficient way to capture patient data. The telephone is time consuming (costly) and relies on accurate transcription over the telephone. The electronic search reveals effective date, waiting period, fiscal or calendar plan year, family members covered by the plan, deductible, maximum, and other relevant information. The electronic search takes less administrative time than the telephone, doesn't rely on memory and handwritten notes, and provides an audit trail. Accurate benefit information is important for both the member and the dentist to make informed decisions. Communication is a key.

Electronic predetermination occurs after the treatment plan presentation but before the treatment date. Except for emergency care, dental treatment need not be delivered on the day of the consultation. The time between the treatment plan and treatment date is usually sufficient to predetermine the dental benefit. When done electronically, the preponderance of procedures automatically adjudicates in seconds without a human eye looking at the claim. Even when the predetermination routes for review or requires additional information, the claim is usually adjudicated in time for the first appointment. The critical piece of the predetermination process is that it is submitted electronically with electronic attachments. Eliminate the need to print a claim, pack it, and post. The electronically predetermined claim sets up the financial arrangement discussion.

Electronic claim submission follows immediately after completion of treatment. The predetermined treatment for is signed, dated, and submitted electronically. There is no need to rekey treatment information.

Direct deposit is the final electronic link in the claim process. The electronically submitted claim takes seconds to adjudicate (it's been predetermined), the money should be in your bank account overnight, and you are alerted to the transaction. Check reconciliation and the explanation of benefits (EOB) are available online.

Electronic dental record (EDR) takes a thoughtful approach because of the cost to implement and maintain. The EDR is primarily thought of as a financial record and dental claim billing system. But the promise of the EDR is more than bookkeeping. There is no excuse to remain in the paper chart world. The competitive small private practice delivers streamlined, patient-centered, cost-efficient care through a series of electronic tools including the EDR.

The next competitive step for the small private practice to take goes beyond the baby steps. There is only so much efficiency that can be derived from a one-man show, where time and resources are limited. Taken separately, recommendation to streamline a practice is easy. But, taken together, all the steps to streamline a small dental practice is impossible. Is there any small dental practice fully compliant with OSHA, HIPAA, employment law, credentialing, and a number of local, state, and federal compliance regulations? Is there any small dental practice willing and able to implement and manage the myriad of excellent business, practice, workflow, marketing, advertising, and human resource recommendations? It seems a self-employed dentist in a small dental practice imposes on themselves working hours and conditions that would be illegal if imposed by an employer. A dentist exploits the dentist labor force at will because the labor force consists of them. Even then, there is never enough time for a small practice owner to address all these issues and treat patients too. The next two steps don't ask you to tinker with the small practice model but ask you to make a fundamental change in how you work.

First, and this might be a baby step too, think at the margin, the cost to produce one additional unit. If a practice is under capacity, the cost to produce one extra restorative procedure is almost zero, and any revenue generated from that procedure goes straight to the bottom line. The practice has already paid for the time. Marginal expense versus marginal revenue analysis is commonly used in manufacturing, for example, the first widget costs $1 to produce, but the 10,000th widget costs 1¢ to produce in the same factory; it is applicable to dental care pricing and forecasting. However, a small practice at capacity may take a financial hit if it changes its existing reimbursement mix when it joins a PPO. The California Dental Association offers models of dental practice that illustrate how this works.

Second, if you believe that a dentist-owned and dentist-operated private practice is the best way to deliver dental care, then the next step takes a leap of faith. The next step is to partner up with a colleague who shares a similar practice style or, better yet, group up with multiple dentists to reach the optimal level for the current facility.

When a dentist thinks about money, they think of the accounting equation "revenue less expense equals income." When income is squeezed, the inclination is to raise revenue. This means to charge higher fees or perform more services. Small private practice is all about raising fees to maintain income. Partnership and groups offer a different solution to maintain income when revenue is constrained, that is, to spread the fixed expense of operation over a wider footprint.

Group practice

Group practice is the way dentists can remain profitable and relevant to dental care delivery. This requires the individual dentist to embrace collaboration and teamwork with other dentists, traits not often associated with dentists. Group practice controls capital investment for a positive return on investment (ROI). Group practice invests in the junior dentist and assures a smooth exit strategy for the senior dentist. The specialist preceptor group model is an innovative way to extend specialty care. Establishing a dental group can occur at any stage of a career but requires an integrator to step up.

Students select dentistry and dental school because the profession offers autonomy as the owners of a small business and comfortable living, not a far-fetched dream but the reality for the dentists who entered practice in my graduation year. A 2015 business magazine ranked dentist as the number one best job out of top 100 jobs. But it's clear that the small private practice is harder to establish and harder to maintain than anytime in the past. The percent of employed dentists grows year-over-year, and they remain employed for a long period of time.

The solution for many dentists in small practice that solves the decline in revenue is to join with other like-minded practitioners in a small group practice arrangement to distribute administrative duties into manageable segments, expand operating hours, and spread the overhead expense over a larger footprint. Thomas Swain is a Denver, Colorado, general dentist who made this happened in his 35th year of practice. Today, he is the managing partner in a dental group and the practice is bursting at its seams with new patients every month (Box 9.1). The point of the Swain model is that a fundamental change practice model can occur at any point in a career. Dr. Swain was in his 35th year of practice when he moved

Box 9.1 My View: Solo to Group

Thomas Swain

Shortly after graduating from Case Western Reserve University in 1971, I opened my solo general practice. Along the way, in 1994, I joined my longtime colleague to purchase a dental building. We maintained distinctly separate dental practices and shared some common space. Thirteen years later, in 2007, we determined that we could achieve better use of our building if we merged practices. And so we did and 4th Avenue Family Dentistry was created. We decided to bring in an associate dentist and knew that in order to keep the new associate busy, we would have to feed him overflow patients and also sign him up to a PPO network. Within 6 months of joining our group practice, our new associate, Chad Braun, built a profitable practice.

The next year, the senior partners joined the same PPO network when it became evident to me that the secret to a profitable practice was to keep patients in the chairs 9 h a day, 5 days a week. The PPO networks provided the number of patients we needed to accomplish this goal. My partner and I shared administrative duties and divided them according to our leadership strengths; I did infrastructure projects like our information technology (IT) system, and my partner did human resources and managed the staff. This division of labor allowed us to distribute multiple administrative duties of a small business to keep it running smoothly while we continued to treat a full complement of patients.

In 2012, 5 years after starting 4th Avenue Family Dentistry, we had grown to the point where we brought into the practice our second associate dentist. The senior dentists arranged their schedules to allow both associate dentists to carry the bulk of patient care leaving time for us to travel without the worry of the practices' viability and continuity of care. Both associates are on track to become partners and owners.

Our success is made possible because our cadre shares a common practice philosophy and believes in the maximal use of our facility. We are hygiene driven with 31 days of hygiene each week. Our recall percentage is 70% and we work to maintain that percentage. We now accept over 150 new patients each month, and most of them have a PPO benefit plan. We don't need chart storage since we converted to an entirely digital format and we plan to convert it into another operatory to enable us to continue to see more new patients. Our overhead is about 50% due to good process management and fully occupied chairs. All of us enjoy the practice of dentistry, and we provide conservative dentistry with equitable incomes for our staff and ourselves.

My key milestones were to form a partnership 20 years into practice and a group practice 35 years into practice. I believe in my colleagues and our group practice model. I just wonder why it took me so long to change.

Reproduced with permission from Thomas Swain. © 2015.

to group practice, and the associate Chad Braun (Box 9.2) was in his first year of practice when he decided to join a group rather than start a solo practice. Both decisions required a leap of faith.

The world doesn't revolve around dentistry and the dental practice. Change, growth, and sustainability only occur in the presence of vision and the absence complacency. Change requires an actionable plan and concerted action. The action can be proactive to remain viable and competitive in the face of change or defensive in the face of a dwindling practice and patient base. In Dr. Swain's case, it is an offensive strategy.

Box 9.2 My View: Associate to Owner

Chad Braun

Upon graduating from Creighton University in 2007, I had four private practice options and decided that 4th Avenue Family Dentistry was the right fit for me. Thomas Swain cofounded a successful partnership that became 4th Avenue. The partners saw the opportunity to bring in an associate in order to begin to accept new patients with PPO dental plans, expand their patient base, and grow the practice. Prior to bringing in an associate, the partners had never before been participating dentists in any PPO provider network.

The partners struggled with the thought of accepting PPO fees that were lower than they were accustomed. I offered them a solution to their conundrum. But if I were to be an asset and not a drag on the office, I would need to build my own practice base. I felt confident in building my practice knowing that two well-respected dentists are my mentors. During the growth period, the partners transferred to me many of their new patients and their incomes surely took a hit. But it sustained me and gave me confidence as my practice grew much more quickly than our projections, and I began to pull my own weight within 6 months. The partners saw, firsthand, the benefit of my participation in the PPO network. Our stable income was made possible by lower operational expense per unit that more than offset the lower PPO fee. My patients were able to afford the necessary treatment, and I was able to deliver the care without any change to my pattern of practice.

Now, having been in the practice for 7 years, I continue to be a proponent of group practice and the PPO network. We continue to grow patient traffic, revenue, and income, because group practice provides an expense to revenue ratio of 55% and the marginal revenue is high. Our group practice has more than 8000 active patients on the books and averages 140–200 new patients per month. My partners (I'm now a partner) and I like being busy, and we like offering a variety of services at a reasonable rate. In addition, our practice predetermines treatment electronically and receives most of our payments the next day when we use electronic claim submission and direct electronic funds transfer to our bank account. It's a relief to be able to concentrate on patient care.

Every year that I practiced, the group's production and collection increased substantially. Most of this success is attributed to the senior partners' vision, focus on spreading expense over a large footprint, and patient growth through PPO participation. In 2013, we expanded and added another operatory that now brings us up to nine. In 2007, we utilized six operatories and now have all nine running 9 h from Monday to Thursday and 7 h on Friday. Currently, we are constructing operatory number 10 from an unneeded chart filing room. We maximize the use of our available space and keep our overhead well below the national average. Our next challenge is, because we are bursting at the seams, we must decide between expanding beyond our four original walls or stop accepting new patients. As they say, a good problem to have.

Thanks to the senior partners' vision and their faith in me, our group practice thrives, and our goal continues to be constant improvement of our comprehensive care model.

Reproduced with permission from Chad Braun. © 2015.

Specialist group practice

An unexplored group practice niche is the pediatric dentist preceptor model. To specialize in pediatric dentistry requires 2 years of rigorous education and training beyond dental school. In practice, the pediatric dentist is the primary care

Box 9.3 My View: Disruption in Pediatric Dental Care

David Okuji

The rub is that there are not enough pediatric dentists to provide care for the children who will acquire dental benefits through the Affordable Care Act.

The nub is that the utilization of general dentists in a pediatric dental specialty practices is a disruptive innovation in dental care delivery whose time has come.

In 2004, the American Academy of Pediatric Dentistry examined the dental workforce issues and correctly predicted that the shortage of pediatric dentists exacerbated by geographic maldistribution would reach crisis proportions in the 21st century. The Healthy People 2020 reminds us that access to dental care by low-income children remains a major public health challenge. The Senate Committee on Health, Education, Labor, and Pensions warns that we must train more oral health providers to treat low-income populations.

To mitigate the rub of a shortage of pediatric dental specialists in an era of increased demand for pediatric dental services, I propose a disruptive innovation to serve as a partial solution. Why not embed general dentists within pediatric practices with the pediatric dentists serving as preceptor and mentor? Historically, the preceptor model for the education and training of dentists was the norm, not the exception, and the pediatric dental residency is a relatively recent event. With the revival of the preceptor model, a pediatric dentist can expand their capacity to care for children by having the general dentist manage the care for children who require routine care. Some have referred to this as the military model of care, where the senior officer oversees and is responsible for the junior officer and all the care within the facility. The pediatric dentist is responsible to credential, calibrate, train, monitor, and evaluate the general dentists. It's expected that all young children squirm, but not all children require a specialist. The pediatric dentist preceptor model frees the pediatric specialist to do what specialists are trained to do: sedation, protective stabilization, interceptive orthodontics, hospital dentistry, and care for patients with special health-care needs.

The call to action to address the shortage of pediatric dentists was heard by organized dentistry. The American Academy of Pediatric Dentistry provides continuing education for pediatric dentists and general dentists who treat children. The California Dental Association Foundation, in collaboration with the California Society of Pediatric Dentistry, established the Pediatric Oral Health Access Program that was designed to help general dentists to become comfortable in treating younger children with an intensive training format.

But short-term courses are not enough. General dentists must be brought into the pediatric care system early in their career and given proper training with continual mentoring in order to deliver appropriate and effective care with confidence. The pediatric dentist preceptor model is especially attractive to general dentists who don't wish to own a practice or practice full-time. The disruptive innovation of the pediatric dentist preceptor model increases the dental system's capacity to treat children and increases their access to care in a dental home. This is a triple win: one for the patient, one for the dentist, and one for the profession.

provider for children with the skill to address complex problems in the office and the operating room. They are supremely capable to address the dental care of children. The rub is there are just too few pediatric dentists to go around. The American Academy of Pediatric Dentistry lists less than 6000 active members in the USA.

One proposed solution is the pediatric dentist preceptor model (Box 9.3). In this model, the pediatric dentist is the leader of a group of general dentists who trains, calibrates, monitors, and directs patient care by the general dentists. They practice in the same facility. The general dentist treats children within their scope of care under the auspices of the specialist and becomes good at delivering that care. The pediatric dentist treats those children that truly require the skill of the specialist. The premise is that the general dentist can appropriately and adequately treat most children if they are properly trained and managed. The pediatric dentist now becomes the manager of a population of children and is responsible for their care and dental health outcomes. This is a new role for a dental specialist in a group practice.

Permanente Dental Associates

Permanente Dental Associates (PDA) of Oregon is a professional corporation formed in 1974 that is owned, governed, and managed by over 100 shareholder dentists. PDA is a group practice with a decidedly different twist on the group model that has promise for the future. PDA is a pure group practice dental delivery play. PDA doesn't own a dental facility. It works out of facilities owned, maintained, and managed by Kaiser Permanente Northwest that is the only Kaiser Permanente region to provide dental services. PDA doesn't own its patients. It contracts with the Kaiser Foundation Health Plan to operate the Kaiser Permanente Northwest Permanente Dental Care Program that delivers dental services to over 180,000 members in Oregon and Washington. PDA is a pure play dental delivery group that can focus on issues like evidence-based treatment, quality of care, practice patterns, medical–dental integration, and population outcome. A pure play dental delivery group can provide dental services to a number of entities including community health centers (CHCs), employer groups, and other hospital systems.

Dental group productivity

Each partner contributes to increased productivity when they focus on management areas of interest or strength. In the case of the Swain model, one partner managed staff and human resources and the other partner managed the information systems and dental technology. To operate a dental practice is a business that must comply with HIPAA, OSHA, IRS, state board licensing, city and state regulation, employment law, provider credentialing, and countless others. The distribution allows the group to comply with multiple rules, laws, and mandates that are mandatory and can't be delayed or ignored. It's the cost of doing business. A solo dentist has limited time available to address these, and the issues are often neglected.

Group practices are open for business more days and hours than a small practice. This results in maximal ROI and provides access to their patients. The group practice increases its income when it maximizes the number of chair hours available per fixed cost and increases revenue through maximizing patient utilization. Small practices are notorious for their short workweek. The 4-day week is a typical with weekend, and evening hours are rarely available on a consistent basis.

These hours force the small practice to spread full-time expense over a part-time base. The small dental practice is open less hours than any other business or profession. It's the wonder of the rest of the labor force.

Whether it's a dental group of three in one facility or six in two facilities, dental group practice offers a number of solutions for dentists to control their own destiny.

Group practice system

Group practice system possesses the structure, process, and financial infrastructure necessary to make a quantum leap in dental care delivery. But, in spite of this robust structure that promises innovation, their operational model remains much the same as the traditional practice. That is, a group practice system is a solo private practice on steroids. It delivers the same service in pumped-up dental offices, by providers practicing like in a solo practice, to the segment of the population targeted by the solo practice. There is very little to differentiate the group practice system from solo practice in execution, price, accessibility, quality of care, patient centeredness, and outcome of care except the capital to open more facilities.

This section suggests that the future competitive advantage for the group practice system is to leverage their strengths to create innovative enterprises: rebrand, off-brand, integrate horizontally, integrate vertically, spin-off services, and new services.

For this section, I refer to a group practice system as a network of multiple offices with multiple dentists as owners or employers that is financed and administered by a dental support organization (DSO). They are systems because the offices are interconnected and share a common vision and mission. They are systems because functions and capital flow freely between each entity. They are systems because of enormous capital resources with one DSO reporting a $1.3 billion capital infusion from a Canadian teachers' pension fund. Each group practice system has a different business model and targets different markets. While one dental group system has a single dentist owner, another dental group system has multiple dentist owners. One system is blue collar focused with a central denture laboratory. Another system focused on consumers with more disposable income prominently displays a CAD–CAM milling machine through a Plexiglas window into the reception area. At the end of the day, they are all dental group systems of the like never experienced in our dental care delivery history and with the promise to change how dental care is delivered: from Joe's pharmacy to Walgreens.

Corporate practice of dentistry

At the turn of the 20th century, legal decisions precluded the emergence of for-profit medical care delivery corporations and ruled that they could not engage in the practice of medicine even if they employed licensed physicians. Respectable

Table 9.1 Dental management service companies (1998).

Company	Headquarters	Ticker symbol
Orthodontic Centers of America	Ponte Vedra Beach, FL	OCAI
Apple Orthodontix	Houston, TX	AOI
Coast Dental Services	Clearwater, FL	CDEN
Dental Services of America	Miami, FL	FLOS
Gentle Dental	Vancouver, WA	GNTL
Monarch Dental	Dallas, TX	MDDS
Princeton Dental Management	Hoffman Estates, IL	PDMC
Castle Dental	Houston, TX	CASL
First New England Dental Centers	Boston, MA	MOLR
OrthAlliance	Torrance, CA	ORAL
Omega Dental	Acton, CA	OMGA
American Dental Partners	Wakefield, MA	ADPI
Birner Dental Management Services	Denver, CO	BDMS

opinion did not favor the corporate practice of medicine over the autonomous private practitioner. The autonomy of the medical professional remained paramount.

The same sense of professional autonomy exists for dentists, and the primacy of private practice in their heart remains unchanged. Access to dental care is held tightly through the professional's hegemony, and private practice was king. Max Schoen's prepaid group practice in Harbor City, California, wasn't well accepted in the 1950s. Neither was a New Zealand-style dental nurse program nor any kind of midlevel provider. However, in the last decade of the 20th century, the hegemony of dentists over dental care delivery was challenged as the corporate model of dentistry came on the scene. In the 1990s, private equity capital, with the prospect of an initial public offering (IPO) payday, fueled the dental corporation roll-up strategy that consolidated individual dental practices into a single entity. In this dental model, companies purchased the assets of existing dental practices—usually larger offices owned by a single dentist—and rolled them up into a single entity to be offered in an IPO on the US public stock exchanges. The roll-up company characterized itself as a dental management service organization (DMSO) to skirt the prohibition of the corporate practice of dentistry. Gasper Lazzara's Orthodontic Centers of America (OCA) was the first dental management service company off the mark and to the market in 1994 as OCAI on the NASDAQ exchange. Other dental roll-up companies followed, and their ticker names appeared on stock market exchanges (Table 9.1). The publicly traded dental practice management company stock price soon stalled when it became apparent that the promised efficiencies of scale and ensuing easy profit were not realized. To merge dental practices with disparate operating systems, cultures, vision, and owners was not the road to riches. OCA moved from the NASDAQ to the New York Stock Exchange (OCA) before it was delisted in 2005. Except for

American Dental Partners and Birner Dental Management Services, the other companies were soon delisted too. Some DMSO names persist today like Coast Dental Services, Castle Dental, and Monarch Dental. Castle and Monarch are under the Smile Brands umbrella.

DSO

However, in the ensuing decade, the DMSO reemerged with a new model and a new name, the DSO. The new iteration DSO built their dreams around de novo rather than roll-up offices. De novo dental offices promised operational efficiency because they overcame the drag of built-in inertia in a roll-up. To build new facilities with new ownership and supported by centralized services with consistent operations, processes again offered the promise of efficiency and profit. In this round, dental workforce recruitment was made easier by the concurrent trend of exploding dental school debt that guaranteed a robust supply of recent graduates needing a job. Dental graduates began to think of employment as more than a stopgap solution in a professional career.

DSOs are well capitalized with one reporting a $1.3 billion-dollar infusion from a teacher's pension fund (Table 9.2). DSOs have a significant brick-and-mortar presence and comprise over 10% of dental locations and access points in some states. DSOs actively lobby to influence dental practice laws favorable to their working model like the passing of the 2011 Kansas dental franchise law. The industry's trade association is the Association of Dental Support Organizations (ADSO) that lists 30 US DSO members in 46 states and a number of industry partners. The California Dental Association is an ADSO member.

Competitive advantage

With the strengths of dental group systems, it's not a stretch to imagine the many directions they can pursue to maintain their momentum, grow beyond their vision, and influence the direction of dental care delivery in ways never before imagined.

Table 9.2 Private equity investment.

Company	Year	Company	Investment
Heartland Dental	2012	Ontario (Canada) Teacher's Pension Plan	$1.3 billion
Smile Brands	2010	Welsh, Carson, Anderson & Stowe	$762 million
Aspen Dental	2010	Leonard Green & Partners	$538 million
American Dental Partners	2012	JLL Partners	$398 million
Western Dental Services	2006	Court Square Capital Partners	$380 million
Kool Smiles	2011	Friedman Fleischer & Lowe	Not disclosed
Mountain Dental	2011	Friedman Fleischer & Lowe	Not disclosed
DentalOne Partners	2008	MSD Capital (Michael Dell)	Not disclosed
Affordable Dentures	2008	American Capital	Not disclosed

Rebrand

DSOs will pursue a strategy to move from a price to nonprice value image to achieve the market position of the trusted source. The shift is accomplished with the emphasis on quality and ethics rather than low price. The market perception pursued is that you can trust us and you won't be oversold; we deliver the right treatment in the right amount at the right time for the right price. No more damaging US Senate reports and Office of the Inspector General (OIG) sanctions. Rebranding is critical to the growth of the DSO model. To drive rebranding, DSOs will recruit a different breed of dental leader. Instead of the clinical expert, they will now recruit leaders in organized dentistry and dental benefit companies who bring a market- and patient-centered view to the enterprise. This flight of talented leadership to DSOs sends a clear signal to the consumer that they are the trusted source.

Off-brand

Each DSO has a specific market niche that they target and a brand they want to protect. But with such a robust infrastructure, there is opportunity to expand beyond the brand. The DSO infrastructure, the back office, has ample capability to develop an off-brand to service new markets. The opportunity to off-brand is especially attractive if multiple DSOs in the same region cooperate to finance facilities and integrate administrative services, marketing, and workforce expertise. Attractive segments to off-brand are the Medicaid, Medicare, and CHIP markets. The child patient market is especially attractive considering the ACA and Medicaid expansion. A DSO's off-brand can be to establish a CHC where it leverages its experience and resources to drive a sustainable and profitable enterprise. Any off-brand is particularly conducive to a collaboration of regional DSOs that protects their midmarket brand.

Integrate vertically

DSOs have already vertically integrated, to some extent, into a central denture laboratory (Aspen Dental), HMO products (Western Dental), and dental benefit companies (Willamette Dental). Other tactical steps are training centers like dental hygiene schools (ODS College of Dental Sciences), AEGD-like programs, and REIT-like arrangements. Vertical integration is powerful but acquires significantly more heft when horizontal integration of DSOs occurs.

Spin-off service

DSOs have the internal expertise and capacity to process dental claims, hire staff, and maintain training facilities. These are internal services available to affiliated dental practices. But it's not a reach to imagine that these services can be offered externally to nonaffiliated dental offices. For instance, a dental claims spin-off leverages expertise and capacity when it offers dentists in solo practice a dumb terminal that sends dental claim data directly to the DSO that administers the claim from eligibility through direct deposit. A human resource spin-off recruits and trains auxiliary staff that is leased by the solo practitioner.

New service

To expand spin-off services, DSOs are positioned to manage and operate the dental section of a federally qualified health center or CHC. Dental sections typically lose money for a number of reasons. But operated in the manner of Sarrell Dental Center (Alabama), a CHC can turn a profit. DSOs are positioned to enter into school-based or rural health-care delivery through hub-and-spoke or teledentistry technology.

Partnership

The ACA offers ample opportunity for the DSO to form medical–dental partnerships. Accountable care organizations (ACO) (coordinated care organizations in Oregon) are natural partners, where the regional DSO assumes the dental care portion of the ACO. Hospital systems are another natural partner where the DSO, in the manner of PDA Group, provides the professional staff or even the brick and mortar and administration. There is the opportunity for collateral benefits like obtaining exclusive access to their insured or redirection of emergency room dental cases to the DSO that lowers the cost of care to the hospital system.

Dentist training model

DSOs obtain a competitive advantage when they deliver effective and reliable dental care. This means the consumer receives the right care that is performed well every time. To accomplish this, the DSO should adopt a military service-like style of provider deployment. In this style, a senior dentist is the preceptor to the junior dentist in the manner of the pediatric dentist preceptor (see specialist dentist group). The dentist preceptor is responsible for guiding the diagnosis, treatment plan, treatment, recare, and outcome of every junior dentist to facilitate standardized care across all dentists in all locations. In this style, junior dentists provide a circumscribed set of procedures in which they become expert to produce efficient and reliable outcomes. For instance, the junior dentists only move from operative to fixed, to periodontal, to endodontic, to implant when they have mastered it. This style promotes dentist satisfaction because you like what you do well and abhor those that fail.

The patient must adjust to the new style but will appreciate that each caregiver is expert in what they do and not expected to do everything. But they always have their primary care dentist (the dentist preceptor), and the delegate procedures are efficient (fast, smooth) and reliable (good results with few failures).

Hub and spoke

The DSO is well positioned to attract patients in nontraditional access points through the hub-and-spoke features. Access points are the spokes that feed into the dental facility hub. Expanding the number of spokes gives the consumer multiple avenues to reach you. The spokes offer a limited menu of dental services specific to the location. The spokes need not be brick and mortar, and nondentist providers staff the spokes. The key administrative features for every spoke are that dental records are linked to the hub and a teledentistry capability is available.

What are spokes? The retail center comes to mind where it caters to families and offers orthodontic adjustments and preventive services. The Walgreen's or Wal-Mart are spokes that offer off-hour services. Storefront locations are spokes that caters to children. School-based programs are spokes. The bus or mobile van is a spoke that rotates through locations like long-term care facilities, hospitals, and rural areas. The hospital emergency room is a spoke in a medical–dental partnership. The CHC is a spoke. The teledentistry hookup is a spoke that reaches. In short, the spoke touches the consumer wherever and whenever they want to access the DSO hub. The consumer can enter the system at any spoke where their recare is addressed and their emergency problems triaged and possibly treated (loose crown) through teledentistry.

The group practice system is ideally poised and ready to assume the position of leadership in dental care delivery. They will attain a commanding competitive advantage in the profession once they implement a number of tactical initiatives that set loose their potential. The group practice system possesses the access to capital, infrastructure, operations processes, leadership, will, and, most importantly, the vision to assume this leadership. The firm hegemony of the solo dental practice is loosened. When the integrator of the group practice system appears, the model shows promise to become the new normal in the new normal.

Safety Net System (SNS)

The dental SNS is in crisis. Financial constraint and systematic deficiency have put them at such peril that can't complete their mission and fulfill their vision. But rather than put safety net clinics on do not resuscitate (DNR), two competitive advantage recommendations are presented: operations improvement and partnership. The competitive strategies are applicable to both a stand-alone dental facility and an integrated health system. The SNS encompasses both the CHC and the federally qualified health center.

Premise
CHCs operate under considerable financial strain. In Colorado, they derive over 60% of their annual revenue from grants and gifts. Four million individuals had accessed dental services at federal qualified health centers in 2011, and 92% of the 20 million patients seen by CHCs had incomes less than 200% of the federal poverty level.

In the future, consumers select dental providers other than a CHC when they gain private dental benefits through the ACA's health-care marketplace. The selection of dental provider may be based on ease of access and perceived quality of care.

Competitive strategy: Operations
CHCs face a daunting task to address the dental needs of a population not familiar with dental disease, dentistry, and dental care. The value of good oral health is weighed against other life challenges. This task is pushed against the fiscal challenge

to deliver care with limited financial resources. The competitive recommendation is to streamline the CHC operations processes to control expense and optimize utilization. No longer is it acceptable to have a full staff and empty dental chairs.

Airline capacity model

The sight of empty dental chairs in the clinic is a sure sign of operational failure that leads to financial distress and is unacceptable whether it's a CHC or a private dental practice. The Sarrell Dental Center (Alabama) often cites its 90% plus chair occupancy rate as attributed to the seat capacity systems used in the airline industry—apropos since the Sarrell Dental Center CEO's brother is the CEO of American Airlines.

The premise to fill seats is to use all the data at your disposal to forecast utilization and then turn it loose on the dedicated call center. The airline capacity model is an interesting construct from which to model a CHC's operation. We envision the airline (CHC) with an airplane (dental clinic) with seats to be occupied (operatory) to deliver the passenger (patient) to a destination (care). The airline, like the CHC, is a capital-intensive and labor-intensive enterprise with thin profits. The airline matches availability to demand. The airline has seasonal demand. The airline matches aircraft to the destination. The airline leaves revenue at the gate when it flies empty but never wants to be at 100% capacity. Cost per seat mile increases when the plane is under capacity. Airlines don't haphazardly overbook passengers to offset canceled reservations. Data collection and data analysis are essential to keep the airline (safety net clinic) running and profitable.

Airline metrics like load factor, revenue passenger mile, revenue per available passenger mile, yield per passenger, and cost per available seat mile all have analogous metrics at the CHC. For instance, consistently high load is not necessarily desirable as it lowers revenue when it leaves too many passengers (patients) at the terminal. It is misplaced pride when dentists beam about their 1-month waiting list for an appointment.

Competitive strategy: Partnership

The CHC doesn't live in a world apart from the financial system. Economies of scale apply to a CHC as well as a DSO. All the features of service are better served in an integrated setting:

- Today, each individual CHC recruits, trains, and retains its own dental workforce. Flexibility and productivity are increased if that same workforce is available to multiple CHCs and strategically allocated. This is especially true for specialist services. This dental workforce will not rely on volunteer dentists. Every dentist is well compensated with the opportunity for advancement and career growth. The CHC dentists are a dental team akin to PDA.
- The costs of outreach service by mobile van and bus, school-based service, teledentistry, hygienist colocation, and nursing home are more efficiently managed and maintained when the administration and cost are spread over a wider base.

- When a CHC shares a dental IT system across a SNS, the patient isn't tethered to any single CHC location and can access dental care at any CHC location within the SNS because a shared IT system allows every location to see the dental record.

To design and implement an innovative competitive SNS strategy requires a bold integrator to foment innovative change and form partnerships between CHCs and between CHCs and outside parties. The integrator can be a CHC, dental service organization, ACO, independent practice association (IPA), hospital–physician system, or an IT company. A CHC dental partnership can include a shared DSO back-office function. Or the CHC dental partnership can contract with an outside administrator to independently operate the CHC dental clinics: finance and operate with a guaranteed minimum return to the CHC. There is no reason a dental CHC cannot throw off a 9% EBITDA profit.

Competitive strategy: Leadership

The SNS needs a new type of dental leader with a skill set that is distinctly different from what we imagine is required. Having superb clinical skill and a passion is not quite enough. The key feature for the new dental leader is a keen understanding that an efficient and effective operation results in a sustainable program. To understand the importance of systems, data, linkages, partnership, and marketing is a skill not taught or acquired in dental school. So the new dental leader may not be a dentist.

The SNS plays a critical role in the dental care delivery system. The SNS of the future is more than financially sustainable and does not rely on grants and gifts to cover the cost of operations; it is profitable to sustain the mission and deliver on its vision. The SNS adopts data analytics and implements rigorous operational systems within an integrated regional network. This integrated system is patient centered, embraces medical–dental integration, and employs a hub-and-spoke system with multiple access points where the consumer can enter the SNS at any access point.

Organized dentistry

This is the most exciting time for organized dentistry in 157 years. There is opportunity to redefine the organization and its mission. The turbulent times prod professional organizations to assess how to better serve the profession and the public. To balance the two is a particularly delicate balance to achieve unless the view is what's good for the profession is also good for the public. The professional is under siege as it faces shrinking membership as dentists look to other sources for their needs to understand health-care finance, flattened revenue and utilization trends, burgeoning dental school debt, and a complicated regulatory environment. So what are the opportunities for professional leadership that leads to competitive advantage? Organized dentistry has a window of opportunity to define and support the notion of the quality of dental care, develop a teledental system that supports access to rural and frontier areas, integrate services for the small dental practice, and sponsor an IPA.

Quality

Organized dentistry, in all of its institutions, has begun to address the difficult question of quality: What is it? How is it measured? Why is it important? Who gets to know? Who gets to choose? The American Dental Association's Dental Quality Alliance is one influential organization that is addressing quality. The American Academy of Pediatric Dentistry has long published guidelines.

For organized dentistry to take hold and lead in the measurement and analysis of quality goes a long way to further its competitive advantage and remain relevant. However, dentists are procedure bound and experience based. Dentists like to do things based on their personal experience: I know it when I see it. Experiential behavior is enabled by the very nature of a private practice where the dentist works in isolation with no oversight. Experiential behavior exacerbates mistreatment when selective memory vividly recalls a successful case and the praise from a grateful patient and forgets the failed case where the patient never returns.

Going forward, the quality will be diagnosis oriented and evidenced based with the notion that it can be measured and the consumer must have access to this information. Organized dentistry's job is to give its members the tools or someone else will develop their own tools.

The key features of a quality program are embedded in the Triple Aim: appropriate care in the appropriate amount at the appropriate time for the appropriate reason with an appropriate outcome. Patient satisfaction in a patient-centered practice rather than a dentist-centered practice is paramount, and cost-efficient care is a required measure. Quality is a multidimensional, and one definition of quality is the degree to which health services for individuals and populations increase the likelihood of desired health outcomes and are consistent with current professional knowledge. Assessing quality is a three-part process involving the structure of care (is it safe), process of care (is the right thing done at the right time in the right amount), and outcome (did it produce the desired result). Dentists might focus on the crown margin, consumers may focus on their wait time for an appointment or how they are treated at the office or how long a filling lasts, and an epidemiologist may focus on the incidence of disease.

The ACA will promote the use of quality measures on the health-care exchanges. Organized dentistry must be the champion for a consumer-facing quality measure document that consumers can use to take more ownership over their oral health care. The profession has the opportunity to capture the public trust. The power of the dental profession lies in the public's trust of our specialized knowledge and skill that is used for their benefit. Trust in the dentist and the dental profession is the paramount virtue to possess, which is a powerful competitive advantage.

Teledentistry

Organized dentistry can play a role in developing and implementing a teledentistry network. The network fits into a rural and frontier dental delivery network. Technology facilitates this innovation that uses electronic communication and IT to provide or support clinical care at a distance. The scope of teledentistry is limited because dentistry is a surgical—not medical—specialty, but it shows promise to expand the scope of the dental practice through hub-and-spoke networks managed.

Teledentistry raises a few issues that organized dentistry can address. First, the scope and level of the dental care delivered by the nondentist provider in a spoke are governed by state dental law. So what procedure can a hygienist in independent practice perform and be compensated, and does that procedure preclude a dentist from doing the same and be compensated? What procedures will organize dentistry support to be included in the basket of goods? Second, do dental practice allow a patient in eastern Colorado confer with a dentist 50 miles away in western Kansas through teledentistry? Third, teledental consultation involves personal health records viewed through computer lines that creates privacy and confidentiality concerns. Fourth, payment for services where the dentist does not interact with the patient—in a store-and-forward situation—may not be a covered benefit. Fifth, will professional liability insurance policies cover services provided through teledentistry?

Teledentistry offers organized dentistry the opportunity to develop and direct this innovative dental care delivery system that sends the important message that patient access to care and equity are important concerns to organized dentistry.

Integrator: Organized dentistry

With its membership comprised of principally small practice owners, organized dentistry can offer its members services to compete in the new normal. The baby step is a group purchasing organization. The ambitious step is to become the integrator of choice for an IPA. One ambitious step further is to become the integrator of choice for its own dental service organization.

Group purchasing organization

Group purchasing is not new to organized dentistry. Many state dental associations offer professional liability insurance to its members at affordable rates. It's not a stretch to imagine that the same organizations offer to dentists in private practice the services and supplies they regularly use but at negotiated prices. Services can be dental software, payroll and payroll tax, employment and training, OSHA compliance, and many more services they regularly use but are too busy to shop and compare. Supplies can converge on a narrow range of choices like implant systems or a single manufacturer's restorative line of products or just a single full service supplier to increase the discount and service. The group purchasing organization is just one part of a continuum of services in organized dentistry's competitive strategy.

Options for action

Organized dentistry faces daunting challenges in leading its small practice owner members and championing quality of care and equitable access to dental care. If organized dentistry decides not to pursue the competitive strategy described earlier, like a purchasing cooperative, IPO, or DSO, there are four other options for action that organized dentistry to be considered in the face of the sweeping change in dental care delivery brought on by the ACA and Medicaid expansion:

Option 1: To maintain the status quo is a passive response to one of the most important laws to affect the finance and delivery of health care in over 50 years. No one likes a change from comfort, and dentists have been very comfortable in small private practice. One reason to maintain the status quo is to wait and observe how the health-care system learns to adapt to this change. This is not too unusual as the dental profession historically lags a decade or more behind the medical profession in adapting to change. Dentistry followed medicine in its anticipatory guidance, patient safety, patient-centered health-care homes, quality improvement systems, and evidence-based practice. So, maybe, organized dentistry has the benefit of time to adjust and follow lessons learned from the medical profession. A disadvantage to maintaining the status quo is that access to dental care is primarily in private practice that hasn't been up to the mark in widening access to cost-efficient care. Our society as a whole may view the dental profession as not fulfilling its social covenant as a public good. Should this perspective of restricted access to dental care escalate where the benefit ticket is left unpunched, a backlash is likely to occur where the dental profession is seen as uncaring. For example, legislation can be brought forward to mandate that licensed dentists in private accept a minimum number of individuals with Medicaid dental benefits. The Colorado Dental Association's voluntary Take Five program is a step in the right direction but mustn't be viewed legislators as self-serving window dressing. Far from being the safe decision, to maintain the status quo is fraught with danger.

Option 2: To advocate for Medicaid fee increase is a proactive action by organized dentistry but may sound tone-deaf when heard by legislators. Calls by organized dentistry to increase the Medicaid fee schedule have, instead, been met with reductions in fees. In 2013, California reduced the fee-for-service dental reimbursement rates by 10%. Another proposal by organized dentistry is to allow dentists a deduction on their federal income tax return for charity care, the difference between their usual, customary, and reasonable fee and the Medicaid fee. This proposal is unlikely to occur because it diminishes tax revenue, is rife with the potential for abuse, and exposes the dental fee-for-service model as a free-for-all with fees having little relationship to cost accounting.

Option 3: To repeal the ACA as a coordinated action by organized dentistry is a nonstarter. This option requires the coordinated action with other groups, is expensive, and has the premise that all members of organized dentistry agree. To support repeal without an alternative plan to address quality and access is not constructive and smacks of self-serving positioning by an elite profession.

Option 4: To acknowledge and adapt to the ACA is a proactive response that puts organized dentistry at the table. The power of competitive advantage for organized dentistry comes to bear where it supports small private practice in a new configuration that can thrive in the new normal, supports and defines the goal of the Triple Aim in dentistry, provides the capacity to address the needs of the most vulnerable in our communities, creates more business for dental practices, and demonstrates that organized dentistry strives to fulfill the social covenant. The mission statement of the American Dental Association reads, in part, "The ADA promotes the public's health through commitment of member dentists to provide quality oral health care, accessible to everyone." Organized dentistry remains a significant player in dental care delivery when it addresses head-on the hurdles of the ACA and do not accept the status quo.

Integrator: IPA

If small private practice is, indeed, at risk to remain relevant in dental care delivery with other players emerging to nudge them aside, then the IPA structure for small private practice may be one competitive advantage solution for them with organized dentistry as the integrator.

The IPA is a network of independent providers that contract with managed care organizations, employers, hospital systems, ACO, federally qualified health centers, and other entities to provide dental services. The IPA can be integrated administratively, financially, clinically, or all in varying degrees. Members of an administratively integrated IPA share the cost of central systems, members of financially integrated IPA share financial risk, and members of clinically integrated IPA share quality improvement goals. Providers who wish to avoid financial or clinical integration may use a messenger model to convey price information to a payer.

The design and implementation of an IPA requires careful thought and planning in order to pass antitrust scrutiny and not be viewed as per se illegal price fixing. The IPA financial risk sharing and clinical integration should involve sufficient integration to demonstrate that it is likely to produce significant efficiencies that benefit consumers and any price agreements by the network providers are reasonably necessary to achieve those efficiencies. Pay for performance arrangements may constitute a form of financial risk sharing. To determine whether a provider joint venture is sufficiently financially integrated to avoid appearance of illegal per se price fixing, the extent to which a pay for performance arrangement constitutes the sharing of financial risk and the relationship between the providers' pricing agreement and pay for performance is of importance. IPA financial integration creates an incentive for provider members to provide cost-efficient quality care.

IPA clinical integration is aided in some circumstances by asking questions like the (i) use of common IT to ensure exchange of all relevant patient data, (ii) development and adoption of clinical protocols, (iii) care review based on the implementation of protocols, and (iv) mechanisms to ensure adherence to protocols. The clinically integrated IPA may do a better job to monitor and manage patients with chronic illnesses like periodontal disease and dental caries than a single independent practice. Clinical integration allows providers to share information more effectively and can jointly employ a care management team. Population management programs to improve patient care and outcome are a competitive differentiator. The clinically integrated IPA can employ dentists to fill in gaps in service coverage including underutilized facilities, extended hours, and emergency care. The administrative, financial, and clinical integration infrastructure is expensive and provider members must be willing and able to make the necessary investment to their future and the future of the small private practice.

Integrator: IT company

The integrator with the best prospect to be a successful integrator of a dental practice system is in the IT industry. The dental practice system of dispersed brick-and-mortar and alternative access points working in concert with a medical system requires a robust IT system. The dental galaxy is made up of multiple dental delivery access points held together by gravitational attraction, that is, the IT system. Graphically, the dental galaxy has planets that are the dental hubs that are the centers for surgical services in master clinician centers; moons that circle the master clinician centers hubs that provide access points to the surgical centers and postoperative, preventive, and emergency care; and asteroids that are nonaffiliated offices that utilized the certain services of the dental galaxy like dental claim processing service, staff recruitment and training, payroll services, and emergency services. It's the sun, the IT capability, that holds the entire system together because the administrative capability is centralized and dumb terminals are used (i.e., the gravitational pull in this analogy) throughout the system so the processing power of the dental record is available at all sites. The sun also provides a bridge to the medical universe to share data in an integrated medical–dental universe where dental hygienists are colocated in physician practice and a nurse practitioner in the dental galaxy (Figure 9.1).

For the consumer, a robust IT system allows them to select any access point to enter the galaxy. For instance, a consumer will have restorative services at a hub where the surgical expertise is centralized, like the hospital in a medical setting. But once the patient reaches maintenance, they can access any spoke facility (retail, mall, Costco, mobile van, rural center, school-based program) for routine

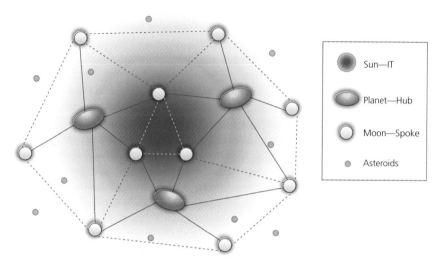

Figure 9.1 IT dental galaxy.

diagnostic and preventive care. In the case of a minor emergency, like a loose crown, a patient in the dental galaxy can access the most convenient hub or spoke for emergency care.

The IT gravitational center attracts nonsystem offices that are not a part of the dental galaxy. These independent offices utilize dumb terminals and the IT dental claim and financial resources to streamline their dental claim operations without a large capital outlay and the ongoing operational maintenance.

The IT integrator solution is the best bet for a successful dental delivery system that delivers patient-centered care with multiple access points with ease of entry, complete scope of services, consistent service, medical–dental integration features, and health outcome focus, which is cost efficient. It will be the dental delivery system of choice for large employers, ACO, and individual consumers that seek consistency that is customer friendly and, above all, trustworthy.

Conclusion

Dentists are not an island entire of themselves, as we like to believe. While the isolated small private practice has been the haven for dentists throughout 20th century, it doesn't seem to be so in the 21st. The best and most cost-efficient care won't necessarily be delivered at the solo practice level.

From the beginning of the new millennium, consumers changed their behavior in regard to access, utilization, and payment for dental services. Consumer visits to the dentist and dentist income flattened after decades of steep growth. Both trends started well before the 2008 recession and are projected to continue into the foreseeable future. The ACA and Medicaid expansion promises wider accessibility to health care and introduces complexity into a health-care delivery system that thrived on procedure-driven care and rising fees.

This chapter suggested strategic visions for different dental care delivery segments that can be reasonably implemented to achieve a competitive advantage. Innovative strategies require an integrator with the will and resources to rationalize the dental delivery system. Strategies that center on IT infrastructure and system integration for the small private practice, group practice, group practice systems, SNS, and organized dentistry are keys to competitive advantage that promises to be sustainable, profitable, and meaningful. The reading of the competitive strategy reveals that each segment of the dental care delivery system is not completely autonomous and housed in a distinct silo. The integrator integrates across all the system silos to give the needed economies of scale to allow each segment to become much more productive and profitable as they achieve their mission. The first-mover integrator's financial commitment and use of dedicated systems erect a formidable, almost insurmountable, barrier to entry. So leadership in the dental care delivery industry just might boil down to who's the first to the party.

The premise of the American free market is that consumer welfare is maximized by open competition and consumer sovereignty—even when a complex health-care service is involved. Competition is dominated by the dental profession whose defense of professional autonomy slows the emergence of alternate solutions to dental care delivery. A procedure-driven system in a fee-for-service payment system rewards quantity of service. A dearth of standardized quality metrics that are routinely measured and reported impedes meaningful dental health outcome goal seeking. The current dental delivery system serves a segment of consumers very well but not the majority. The dental care delivery system is not a system but more controlled chaos for the consumer and payer of dental care.

The tipping point is upon us and more chaos is in the cards before meaningful change is reached. The nature of the triumphant integrator determines the course of dental care. We now move from analysis to action.

Index

Dental Benefits and Practice Management: A Guide for Successful Practices, First Edition.
Edited by Michael M. Okuji.
© 2016 John Wiley & Sons, Inc. Published 2016 by John Wiley & Sons, Inc.